BOBBI BROWN

PRETTY POWERFUL

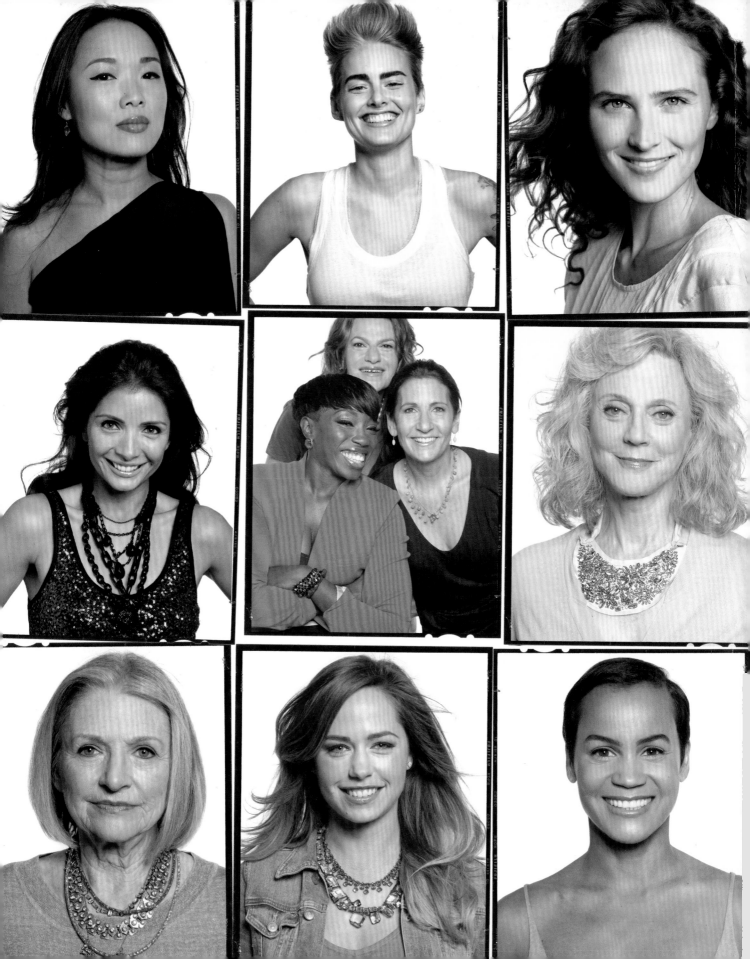

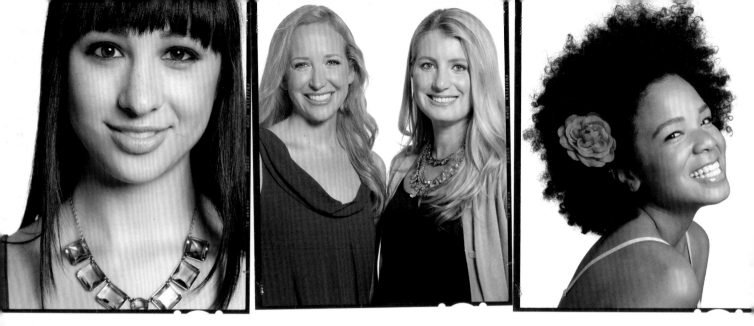

BOBBI BROWN

PRETTY POWERFUL

Beauty Stories to Inspire Confidence
Start-to-Finish Makeup Techniques to Achieve Fabulous Looks

By Bobbi Brown with Sara Bliss

CHRONICLE BOOKS
SAN FRANCISCO

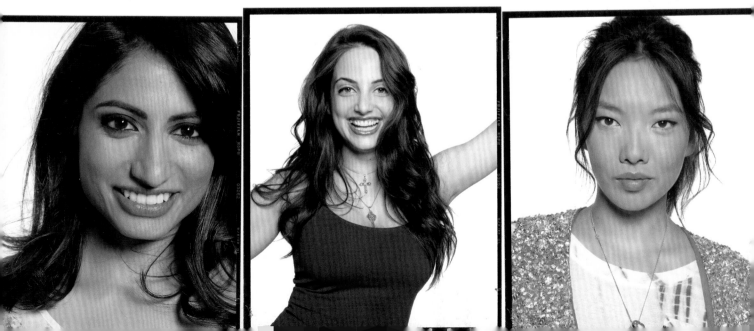

LIBRARY OF CONGRESS CATALOGING-IN-PUBLICATION DATA

BROWN, BOBBI.
   BOBBI BROWN PRETTY POWERFUL : BEAUTY STORIES TO INSPIRE
CONFIDENCE / BOBBI BROWN.
      P. CM.
   INCLUDES INDEX.
   ISBN 978-0-8118-7704-6
   I. BEAUTY, PERSONAL. 2. WOMEN—HEALTH AND HYGIENE. 3. SKIN—
HEALTH AND HYGIENE. 4. SELF-CARE, HEALTH. I. TITLE.

RA778.B6693 2012
646.7'2—DC23

                         2011053149

MANUFACTURED IN CHINA

DESIGNED BY AYAKO AKAZAWA

ABC News is a registered trademark of American Broadcasting Companies, Inc. Bloomingdale's is a registered
trademark of Federated Department Stores, Inc. Boys & Girls Clubs is a registered trademark of Boys' Clubs
of America Inc. Bulgari is a registered trademark of Ditta Sotirio Bulgari di Costantino e Giorgio Bulgari, S.a.s.
Converse is a registered trademark of Converse Inc. eBay is a registered trademark of eBay Inc. Gilt Groupe is a
registered trademark of Gilt Groupe, Inc. Gnu is a registered trademark of Gnu Foods, LLC. Grammy is a registered
trademark of National Academy of Recording Arts & Sciences, Inc. Helen Ficalora is a registered trademark of
Jewelry Boutique, LLC. Kleenex is a registered trademark of Kimberly-Clark Worldwide, Inc. L.L. Bean is a registered trademark of L.L. Bean, Inc. Christian Louboutin is a registered trademark of Christian Louboutin. Louis Vuitton is a registered trademark of Louis Vuitton Malletier. Nike is a registered trademark of Nike, Inc. Proenza Schouler
is a registered trademark of Proenza Schouler, LLC. Spanx is a registered trademark of Spanx, Inc.

10 9 8 7 6 5 4 3 2 1

CHRONICLE BOOKS LLC
680 SECOND STREET
SAN FRANCISCO, CALIFORNIA 94107
WWW.CHRONICLEBOOKS.COM

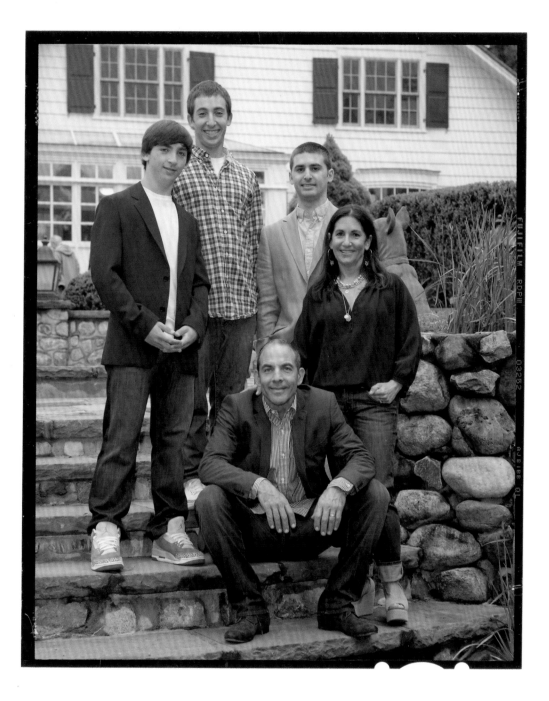

This book is dedicated to all the women in my life who taught me to be Pretty Powerful
and to the boys and men in my life who love me for who I am.

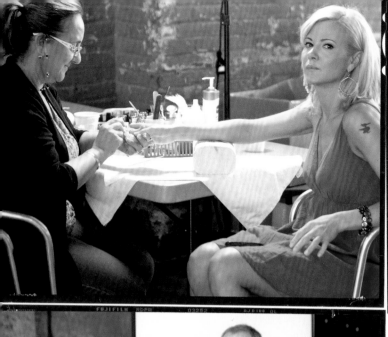
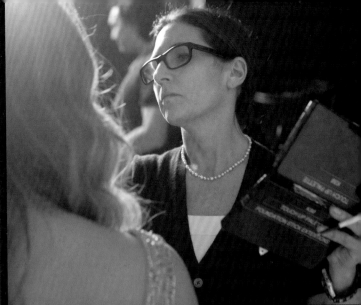
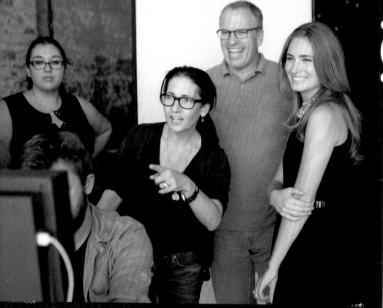
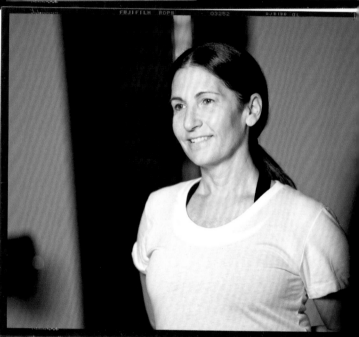
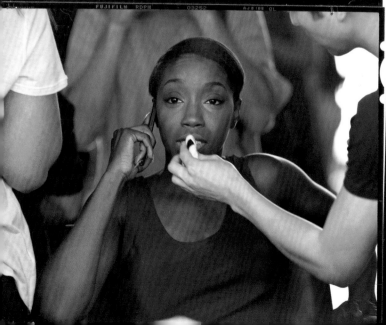
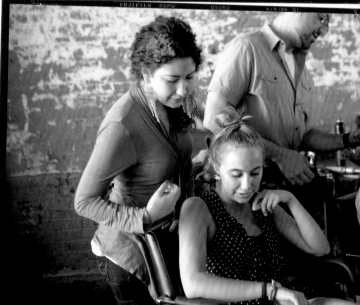

CONTENTS

———

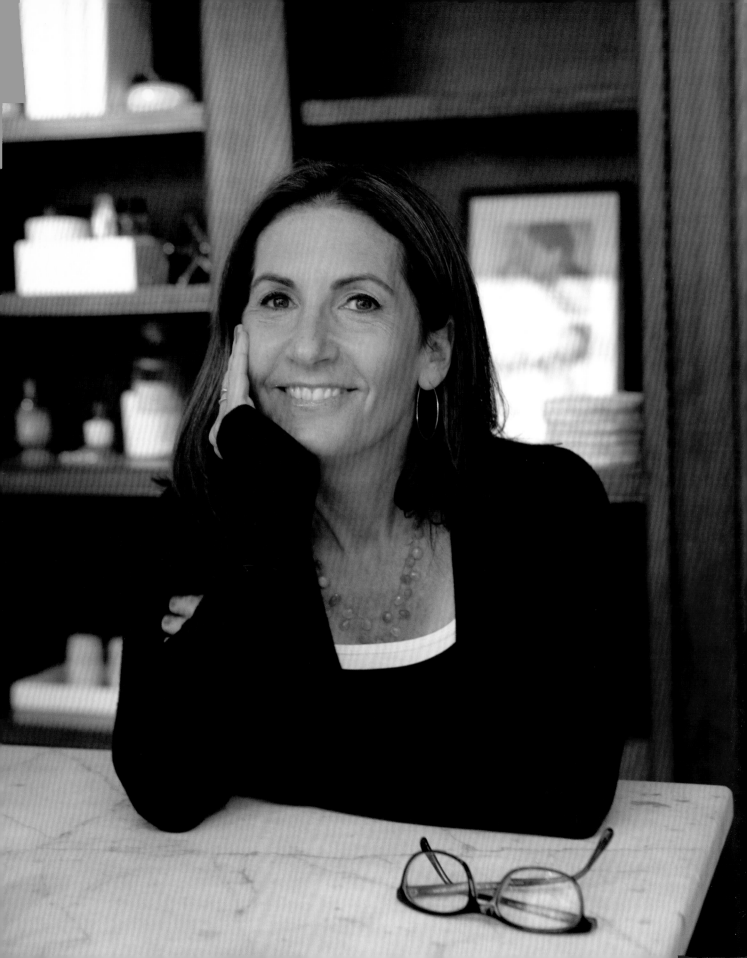

INTRODUCTION

I live in a house of men. Between my husband, three sons, two nephews, and (as I write this) two foreign exchange students (who we fondly call the "Euroboys"), I am definitely in the minority at home. Luckily for me, my two female dogs, Biggie and Pup Pup, are there for cuddling. That's my home life. But in my work life, I am surrounded by women: young ones, old ones, tall ones, short ones, pregnant ones, menopausal ones, and many who don't always feel pretty.

While looking at the "before" photos for my last book, *Beauty Rules*, I had an epiphany. Even though I'm in the business of selling makeup, I loved how the teens and their moms looked without any makeup. But I also loved how everyone lit up after the makeup was applied and the sparkly jewels were put on. The "after" shots were stunning and authentic. The message behind *Pretty Powerful* is simple: All women are pretty without makeup and can be pretty powerful with even just a touch of makeup.

As a makeup artist, beauty expert, and woman, I understand what it takes to feel and look good. It takes an incredible amount of hard work (as does everything that's worth doing)—you have to eat right, exercise regularly, learn how to apply your makeup, and get dressed even on days you're not feeling your best. But first and foremost, feeling good requires an upbeat attitude, confidence, and a wicked sense of humor. And that's what *Pretty Powerful* is all about.

This book is more than gorgeous photos. It's a book about incredible women and their inspiring words. It includes application techniques you can use at home and personal stories that will inspire you to be your best, most authentic self. Creating *Pretty Powerful* was an unforgettable experience; I had the honor of working with an amazing collection of women, each celebrating life and full of energy and confidence. My hope is to help women everywhere understand that being who you are is the secret to lasting beauty—and that all of us can be both pretty *and* pretty powerful.

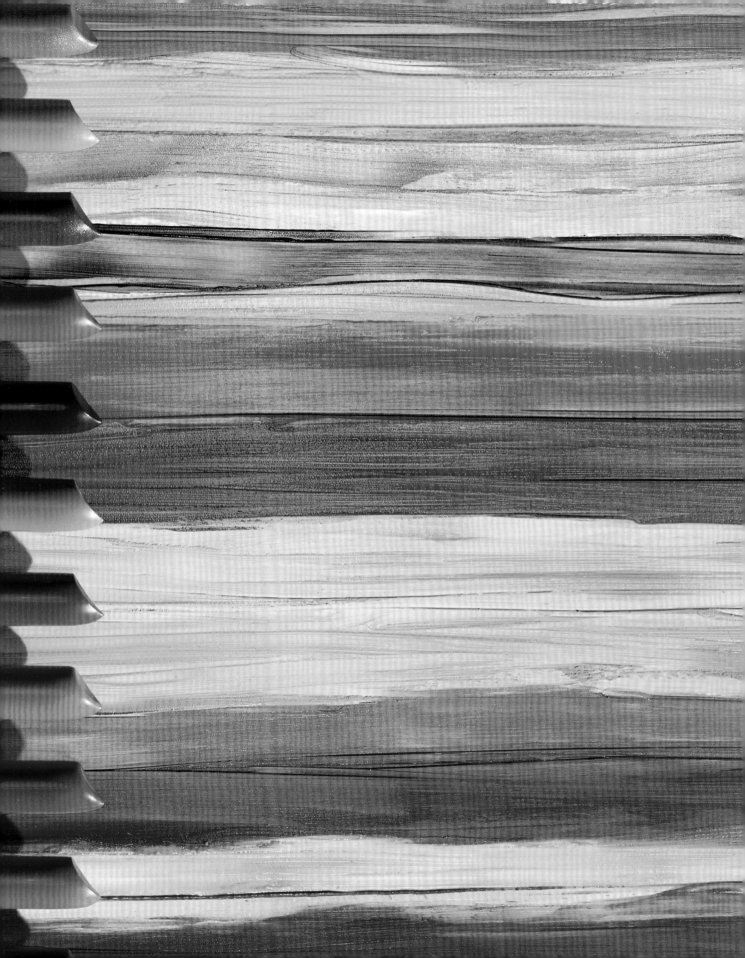

IO-step beauty

MAKEUP BASICS

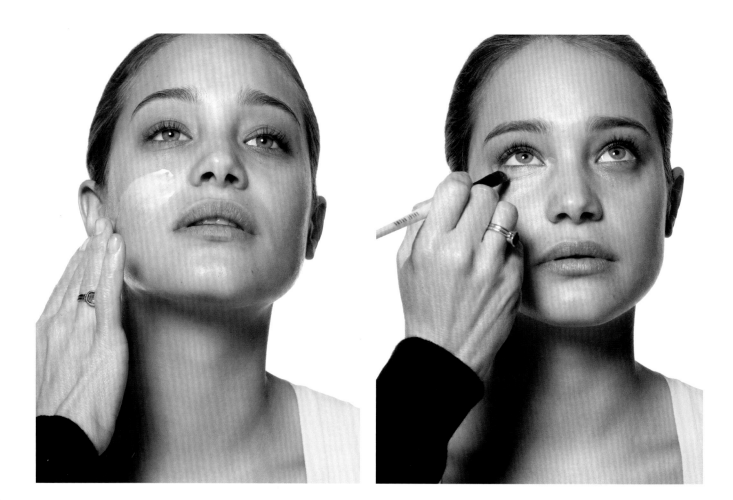

1. MOISTURIZER

Moisturizer is the key to keeping skin hydrated and looking fresh. It also ensures that concealer and foundation go on smoothly and evenly.

When you are selecting a moisturizer, choose a formula for your skin type. You can find moisturizers for all types of skin—oily, dry, combination, normal, or acne-prone. You know you are using the right moisturizer when skin looks hydrated, free of pores, and radiant but not shiny.

In the morning, immediately after splashing your face with cool water, apply the correct SPF moisturizer all over your face and neck. Use a richer nighttime formula to plump up and restore skin while you sleep. Don't forget to moisturize the delicate eye area using your finger to gently pat a hydrating eye cream into skin.

2. CORRECTOR & CONCEALER

For very dark circles or days when you need extra coverage, start with a corrector to brighten and neutralize discoloration under the eyes. Pink tones neutralize pinky-blue darkness, and peach tones neutralize purple-brown darkness. In general, light to medium skin tones should use corrector in pinky-bisque shades, while medium and warmer skin tones should use peach-toned correctors. Use a concealer brush to apply corrector as close as possible to the lash line and also on the innermost corner of the eye. Gently blend the corrector with your fingers.

A yellow-based concealer one shade lighter than your complexion works to brighten the undereye area for all women. If you are using a creamy concealer—a good choice for more coverage—apply it directly over the corrector with a brush and then gently blend in with your fingers. For lighter coverage, a lightweight undereye concealer pen can be applied directly with the built-in brush and then blended with fingers.

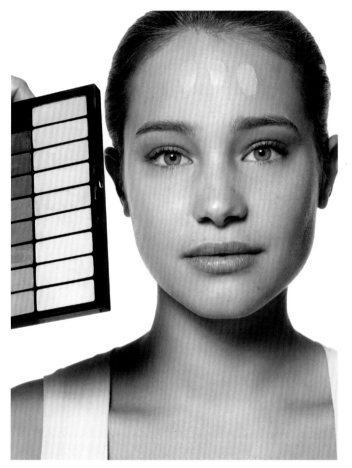
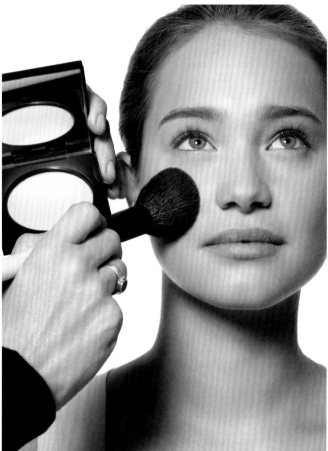

3. FOUNDATION

There are many different foundation formulas to choose from. Whether you prefer the sheer, lightweight texture of a tinted moisturizer, the buildable medium-to-full coverage of a foundation stick, or the breakout-preventing benefits of an oil-free foundation, you can find a formula that is right for you. To choose the correct color, start by trying three shades of a yellow-toned foundation on the side of your face as well as your forehead. (All women have yellow undertones in their skin; a yellow-based version will look the most natural.) The right foundation should look like you aren't wearing makeup at all—so the shade that disappears into both your forehead and your cheek is the right one for you. Make sure you look at the options in natural light.

4. POWDER

Not only does powder give skin a smooth and polished appearance, but it also holds foundation and concealer in place. To apply, use a powder brush, or puff, to cover the skin with a light dusting of loose or pressed powder. Always blow or tap excess powder off your brush so that the makeup doesn't flake on your face as you apply. Choose pale yellow or white powder to apply over undereye concealer, depending on your skin color (choose white if you have alabaster or ivory skin; pale yellow for all other skin tones). For oily skin, concentrate on eliminating shine from your T-zone, across the brow and down your nose and chin. Loose and pressed powder work exactly the same, but I find that loose is better to use at home, while pressed powder is great for on-the-go touch-ups. Stay away from translucent powder because it makes skin look chalky and ashy. Most women look great with a yellow-based powder that matches their skin tone.

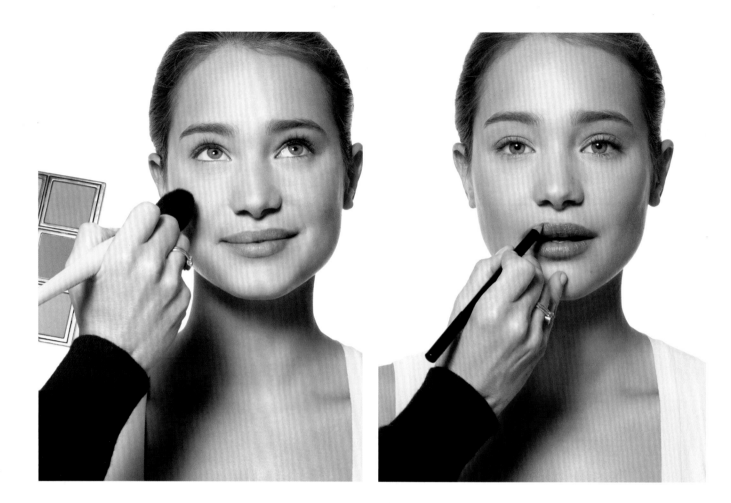

5. BRONZER & BLUSH

To add a healthy warm tint to the skin, dust a bronzing powder over cheeks, forehead, nose, chin, and neck using a bronzer brush. Bronzer is great for countering redness in skin and blending the look of foundation on the face with the neck. Bronzer is best applied with a full, flat brush.

To apply and blend blush, choose a smaller, slightly rounded brush. Smile and dust a neutral shade of blush on the apples of the cheeks. Blend up toward the hairline, then back downward to soften color. For a brighter look, apply a pop of bright blush just to the apples of cheeks. If you are using a pot rouge, take two fingers and dip them into the color, apply to the apple of the cheek, and in a circular motion blend up toward the hairline and back down, rubbing it in for beautiful natural-looking color.

6. LIPS

Use the natural coloring of your lips as a guide when choosing your everyday lipstick shade. The most flattering color will either match or be slightly darker than your lips. This will be your perfect nude lipcolor.

There are many great finishes to choose from when it comes to lipstick. A matte finish lipstick gives a flat, polished finish, and the denser formula tends to last longer. A sheer lipstick offers transparent but pigmented color. Shimmer lipsticks add a touch of sparkle. Gloss brings shine and hydration, giving the lips a fuller, wetter look.

If you want to add lip liner for natural-looking definition, line lips with a liner the same shade as your lipstick after applying lip color. Use a lip brush to soften and blend any hard edges.

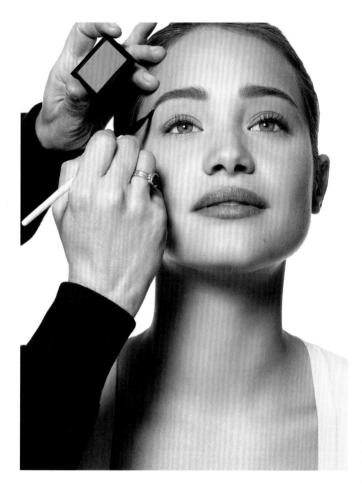

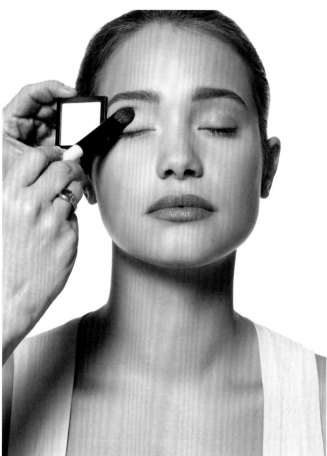

7. BROWS

For the most natural look, define brows with an eye shadow that matches your natural brow shade and hair color. Use a hard slanted eyebrow brush to apply the shadow. Begin at the inner corner of the brow and follow its natural shape using light, feathery strokes. Finish with a coat of clear brow gel to tame brows and provide a polished finish. For the most flattering brow shape, I recommend having a professional groom your brows first and then doing the upkeep yourself at home with tweezers.

8. EYE SHADOW

For a pretty three-step eye, start by sweeping the lightest eye shadow base color from lash line to brow bone using an eye shadow brush. Dust a medium eye shadow color on the lid up to the crease. Lightly sweep the darkest shadow right above the crease and blend in for depth.

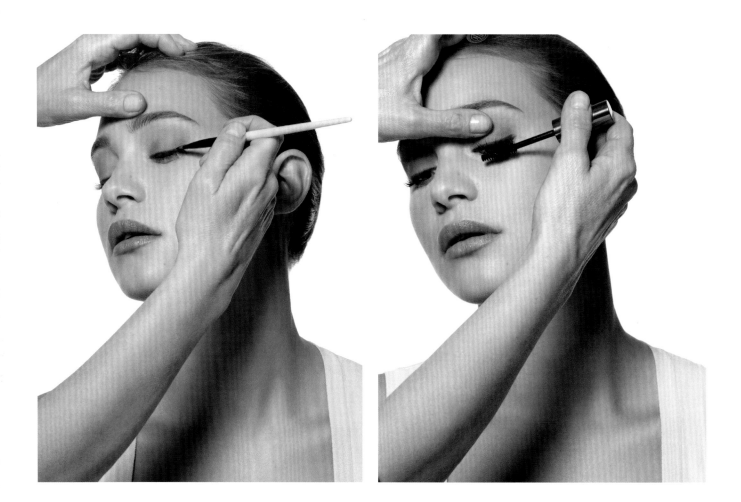

9. EYELINER

Use an eyeliner brush to line the upper lash line with a dark eye shadow color. Start from the outer corner and work your way in, applying the line as close to the lash line as possible. For a longer-lasting look, dampen the brush before dipping it into shadow or try a gel eyeliner for a line that stays put.

If you want your eyes to stand out, also line the lower lash line, making sure that the top and bottom liner meet at the outer corner of the eye. The trick is to have the liner be stronger on the top rim and softer on the bottom to open up the eye.

10. MASCARA

True black mascara makes the most impact; even for blondes it really makes eyes pop. To apply mascara, brush from the base of your lashes to the tips. Roll the wand as you go to separate lashes and prevent clumps. Depending on your preference, apply one to three coats. If you choose to curl lashes, be sure to do this before applying mascara; curling lashes after mascara makes them more prone to breakage. Using an eyelash curler, clamp lashes for five seconds on each eye.

MAKING YOUR MAKEUP LAST

Keeping your makeup looking as good at 4 т.ʊ as it did first thing in the morning is easy. With a few touch-ups and the right formulas, your makeup can look great all day.

——

Choose long-wear formulas that won't fade as easily as standard makeup. Make sure they have at least an eight-hour last.

A foundation stick is compact and allows you to eliminate any redness throughout the day. Use it for touching up places where makeup has worn off.

To keep shine at bay, touch up with pressed powder and a puff. For problem oily areas, choose a mattifying lotion under an oil-free foundation.

To keep a pretty pop of color on the cheeks, layer powder blush over cream blush—or the reverse—to revive color and glow. Be sure to blend carefully.

Lips can be touched up throughout the day straight from the tube. Use a pencil on top of lipstick to make it last longer.

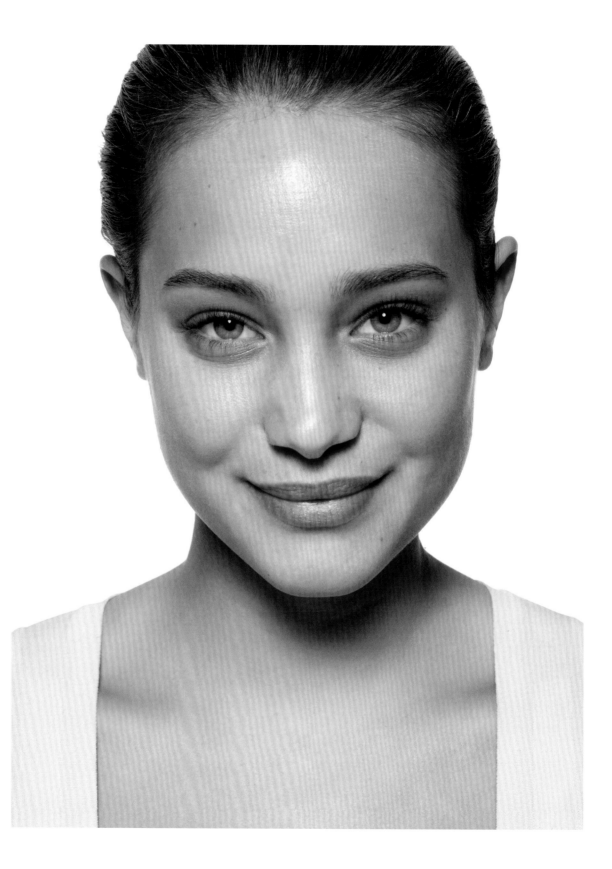

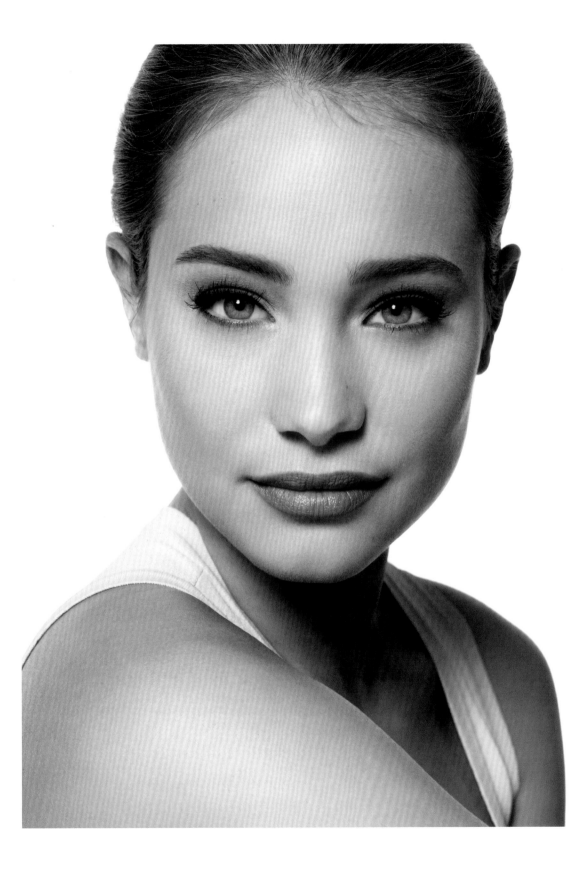

TAKING YOUR MAKEUP FROM DAY TO NIGHT

To turn your daytime makeup into a pretty party-ready look, just go deeper, brighter, or more shimmery.

———

If you normally wear brown eyeliner, switch to black for evening. Black adds drama and glamour.

If you usually wear one coat of mascara for day, go with three for night. To enhance your eyes, go with the blackest mascara you can find. Then curl lashes with your fingers to really open them up.

A little sparkly iridescent shadow on the lower lid looks gorgeous at night— it can also be placed under the eye on the inner corner for subtle drama.

If you often wear a pretty simple eye during the day, try a glamorous smoky eye for night. Add a darker shadow on the lid and smudge up to the crease, blending and adding more to achieve the desired effect.

A touch of shimmer on the apple of your cheeks over your blush is a quick way to illuminate your skin for evening.

Going deeper in color is one way to take lips from day to night. If you wear pinky and rosy tones during the day, try going a shade or two darker for night. If you prefer softer shades, choose a shimmery version for night.

A red or pink bright lip looks best with a cleaner eye and a pastel blush. Light shimmer lips look fantastic with a stronger eye and a pop of brighter blush.

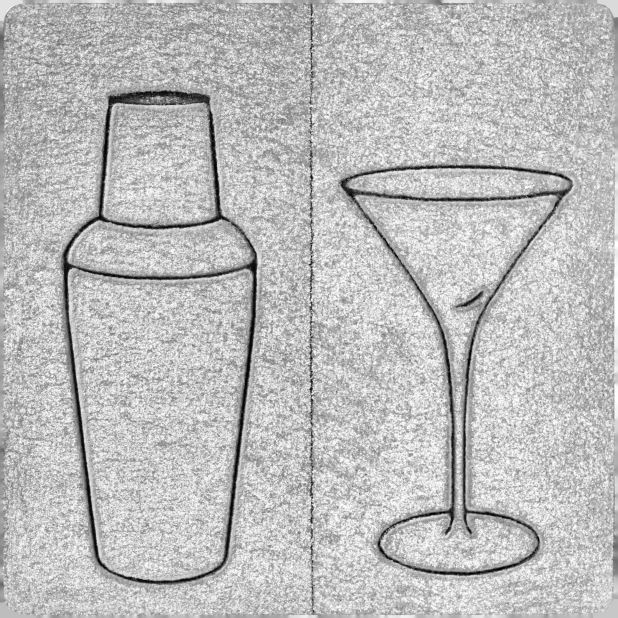

BEAUTY FROM THE INSIDE OUT

It takes work to look and feel your best.

———

EXERCISE

Beauty is about so much more than makeup. If you take care of your body, it shows. Women who regularly exercise radiate confidence and have a fresh, healthy, and beautiful look. There are so many benefits to exercising—it makes your cheeks naturally rosy, calms the brain, gets rid of pain, makes you limber, brings out endorphins, and just feels great. Cardio—walking, spinning, running, biking, or hiking—gives you an immediate rush of energy and vitality that you feel for hours afterward. The bonus is you look great for days. But it doesn't have to be cardio to make an impact. There are two simple yoga moves that help me stretch and feel centered and energized. I like that I can do them anytime I need to, even in my office. When I'm super tired, I shut my door, lay on my back, and put my feet up against the wall. I focus on breathing for five minutes, clearing my brain, and when I'm done I feel refreshed and ready for anything. I also love the downward dog pose that stretches you from the tips of your toes to the top of your head. It is a move that has made me both limber and strong. Exercise is a powerful tool in many ways. My advice is to do whatever you can to be active, even if that means little things like taking the stairs instead of the elevator, parking your car as far from the store as possible, or just walking around the block. The more you exercise, the more you will become addicted to the results. Combined with eating right and getting enough sleep, exercise is the ultimate beauty enhancer.

EATING RIGHT

Like every woman, my days are packed. Between work, my three boys, my husband, and trying to squeeze in a workout, I'm always busy. To give me the endurance to get through even the most hectic days without crashing, I rely on healthful foods to keep me going. There is also the added bonus of how great you look when you choose nutrient-dense foods. Lots of veggies, fresh juices, whole grains, fruits, lean protein, and fiber are all amazing beauty foods. When I eat right, my skin is rosier, my eyes are brighter, and I'm able to maintain my weight. Here's a sample of some of the foods that I eat for fuel, strength, and beauty.

Breakfast

I have a few go-to choices. I either have oatmeal with berries and protein powder, or a piece of high-fiber toast topped with omega-3 eggs. Sometimes I add spinach or broccoli and some goat cheese.

Lunch

I stick with an easy formula that leaves room for a lot of different food choices. You want variety in your diet to get the most amount of nutrients. I eat a mix of some vegetables, some protein, and some carbs. I usually go for soup with salad or a sandwich depending on my hunger level. I try to eat a lot of veggies, and soup is a great way to get them in. I also love a tuna sandwich on nine-grain toast. I'll eat a half with my soup or salad. I am 100 percent against low-carb diets—they are unhealthy and they don't work.

Afternoon snack

I have three go-to afternoon snacks that I love:

- A really crisp apple (green and Honeycrisp are my favorites) with almond butter
- Crudités and hummus or guacamole—the avocado is great for your skin, and veggies provide nutrients
- A cup of tea along with a high-fiber Gnu bar and a hard-boiled egg fills me up and keeps me hunger-free until dinner

Dinner

I have a general formula that works for dinner. I combine a fat, protein, carb, and as many vegetables as possible. I love the freedom of this way of looking at food. It's not a rigid diet, so I have lots of options. I often eat out at restaurants, which makes eating right more of a challenge. To stay on track, I order crudités or a salad with lemon and olive oil dressing as soon as I sit down. (Since I am always hungry upon arriving, ordering fresh veggies as soon as I sit down helps me steer clear of the bread basket.) A healthful dinner option that I love is grilled fish with a touch of olive oil, hold the salt (I'd rather add it myself so I can control the amount). For sides I go with steamed veggies with rice and beans or quinoa.

Beverages

I feel my best when I begin the day with a giant glass of water with lemon juice. I also have a double shot of espresso with a touch of half-and-half. Green tea is the only caffeine I drink in the afternoon if I'm tired because coffee just makes me crash. Throughout the day I drink plenty of water and herbal tea. I am a fan of fresh-pressed juices and I drink them as often as I can. Celery with kale, spinach, cucumber, and parsley is a favorite mix. Any dark green veggie mix will be loaded with vitamins and nutrients. I also love the occasional clean cocktail in the evening. It's either vodka on the rocks with three olives or tequila on the rocks with fresh lime juice. I don't like wasting calories on juice mixers or sodas, so clean drinking it is. At night, Celestial Seasonings Sleepy Time Extra tea calms me down.

10 Percent Rule

If I eat right 90 percent of the time, I find I can indulge the other 10 percent. It lessens the pressure to be perfect (which isn't possible) and lets me enjoy something indulgent every once in a while.

WATER

Staying hydrated is essential. And surprisingly, it is an easy thing to overlook. Women are often so busy taking care of everyone else that we sometimes forget to do the most basic things for ourselves like drinking enough water. You've probably heard by now that drinking eight 8-ounce glasses of water a day should be your goal—but it is hard to keep track of. What's easier for me is having a pitcher of water on hand filled with slices of cucumber or lemon, and drinking often. I try to hydrate before and after exercise as well as before I eat. When you drink enough water, your skin is plumped up and healthy, you flush out toxins, you have additional energy, and it gives you a great glow.

LIFE BALANCE

Let's be honest: Some weeks, balance just doesn't happen. Between work, family, friends, and making time for yourself, there is a lot to juggle. But as much as I work, my family is always my priority. When my kids were little, I always dropped them off at school in the morning and felt lucky on the days I could pick them up. I also found it helpful to plug in school events to my business calendar, so work revolved around important kids' events. I eat dinner with my husband and some part of my family every night, which means I have to say no to invitations more often than I say yes. And I'm okay with that. As long as work gets done, I am really supportive of my employees going to the school play, taking their kids to the doctor, and, in those inevitable moments, turning their attention from work to family. Life is about focusing on what is important.

THE CHANGING FACE OF BEAUTY
Foundation know-how

———

FORMULAS

Liquid

If you're looking for an even, polished finish, liquid foundation is a great choice. There are a variety of different types of liquid foundations to choose from—from light, sheerer versions to really rich, full-coverage formulas. Whatever type of look and coverage you want, there is a liquid foundation for you.

Foundation stick

Easy to use and incredibly versatile, with a texture that works for all skin types, foundation sticks should be a staple in everybody's makeup kit. Use it just where you need it for simple spot application or all over your face when you want complete coverage. Small and portable, foundation sticks are also perfect for on-the-go touch-ups.

Tinted moisturizer

If you prefer a more natural look, go with a tinted moisturizer. Makeup and moisturizer in one, tinted moisturizers simplify your morning routine and leave a sheer finish that is even lighter than a sheer liquid foundation.

Tinted moisturizing balm

A lightweight to sheer foundation, tinted moisturizing balm is perfect for dry, dehydrated skin. The ultra-rich formula provides extra moisture, plumping up skin for a dewy glow.

Compact powder foundation

Powder foundation immediately cuts down shine. It also has the bonus of being easy to apply and blend with a sponge.

APPLYING FOUNDATION

Foundation brush

A foundation brush can be used with any foundation formula, from a stick to a liquid, giving your skin gorgeous, polished, full coverage. It is a terrific tool for applying foundation all over the face.

Wedge sponge

A wedge provides a similar full coverage finish as a brush but works best with liquid formulas.

Fingers

I always recommend using your fingers to blend after applying foundation with a brush or sponge. Just gently press the foundation onto your face, blending it in so that the foundation is invisible on the skin.

Foundation stick

When using a foundation stick, the easiest application is to take the stick itself and apply it directly on your face, rubbing it in with your fingers. For sheerer coverage, apply it with a foundation brush.

CHOOSING THE RIGHT FOUNDATION FOR YOUR SKIN TYPE

Oily

For oily skin, choose an oil-free liquid or powder foundation that won't clog pores. Additionally, mineral powder combats shine and excess oil, making it a smart choice for oily skin.

Dry

Moisturizing formulas, from a rich, tinted moisture balm to luminous moisturizing foundation to a tinted moisturizer, are your best bets for beautiful coverage that also hydrates skin.

Combination

Pairing the right moisturizer for your skin type with the correct foundation formula is the key to dealing with combination skin. Whether that means pairing an oil-free foundation and moisturizer to avoid breakouts or combining a moisturizing foundation with an oil-free moisturizer, it's all about choosing a combination that gives you smooth, even skin.

Normal

Use anything you feel like!

FOUNDATION FOR ALL SEASONS

In the winter you want creamier, richer formulas, switching to lighter and more transparent versions for spring and summer. Your skin tone changes slightly from season to season—even if you don't tan—so you may want to change not only your formula depending on the season, but your foundation shade as well. Use the tips on page 13 to choose the best foundation for you. Thanks to the sun, many women are one shade darker in the summer than in the winter, but it varies depending on your skin.

BOBBI'S RULES FOR FEELING AND LOOKING SPECTACULAR

Be comfortable / Be confident / Be powerful

Be happy / Be active / Be strong

Be smart / Be open / Be nice / Be still . . .

SEASONAL BEAUTY

Just like your wardrobe, your makeup should change with the seasons

———

SPRING

Spring is about shedding layers, going lighter with both texture and color. Look for sheer formulas—a lighter foundation, soft eye shadows, and sheer glosses with a hint of color. Spring eyes are about lighter hues for lids and a soft touch of shimmer. With cheeks and lips you want to use the colors blossoming outside for inspiration. Think pastels, pinks, and peach tones. Spring is the time for bright and pretty makeup.

SUMMER

In summer you don't need a lot to look gorgeous. A little bit of bronzer, a pop of blush, waterproof mascara, a pretty gloss or a pale shimmery lip, and you're ready for anything. Women blessed with beautiful skin can skip foundation altogether. A tinted moisturizer is terrific in the summer. Many versions have SPF, and they simplify your routine. If your skin gets oilier in the summer, look for oil-free formulas; for very oily skin, go with a mattifying foundation with a mattifying lotion underneath. Long-wear and waterproof mascara and gel eyeliner will stand up to heat and humidity.

AUTUMN

Say good-bye to the shimmery casualness of summer makeup and switch to richer tones and denser formulas that will give you a more polished look. Choose a foundation that evens out your skin a bit more. Go for denser lip color in classic fall colors like brown or cognac. For blush, look for warmer shades of dusty pinks or roses. Going from summer to cooler-weather makeup is a little like swapping your airy cotton sweater for a cashmere one—think stronger, richer, and warmer.

WINTER

Holiday makeup is all about sparkle, glitter, and fun. You also need to focus on moisturizing and pampering your skin to cope with the harshness of dry cold months. Switch to richer moisturizers for both day and night to plump up skin. Pick creamier formulas for your makeup, anything with moisture—pot rouge for blush, moisturizing foundations, and hydrating lip gloss. For moist gorgeous lips, you can also try layering moisturizing gloss over creamy lipsticks. You can counteract pale winter skin with bronzer, which instantly warms up your complexion. Two blushes—a natural shade and a pop of something brighter—will give you a natural healthy glow and prevent that pale, washed-out look that hits along with the frost.

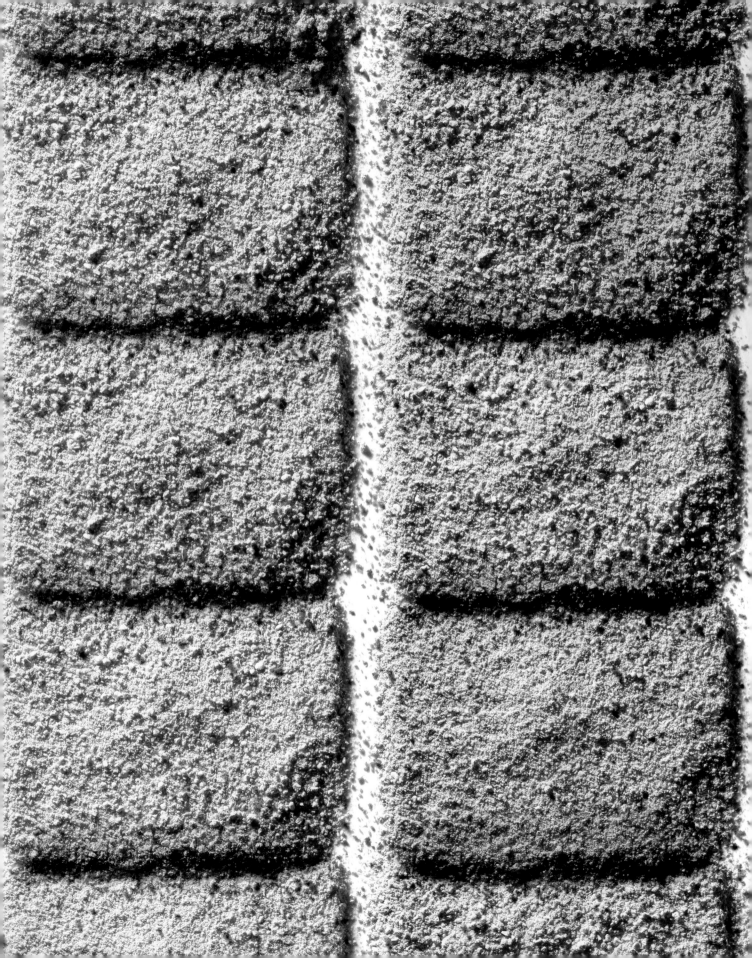

01

PRETTY NATURAL

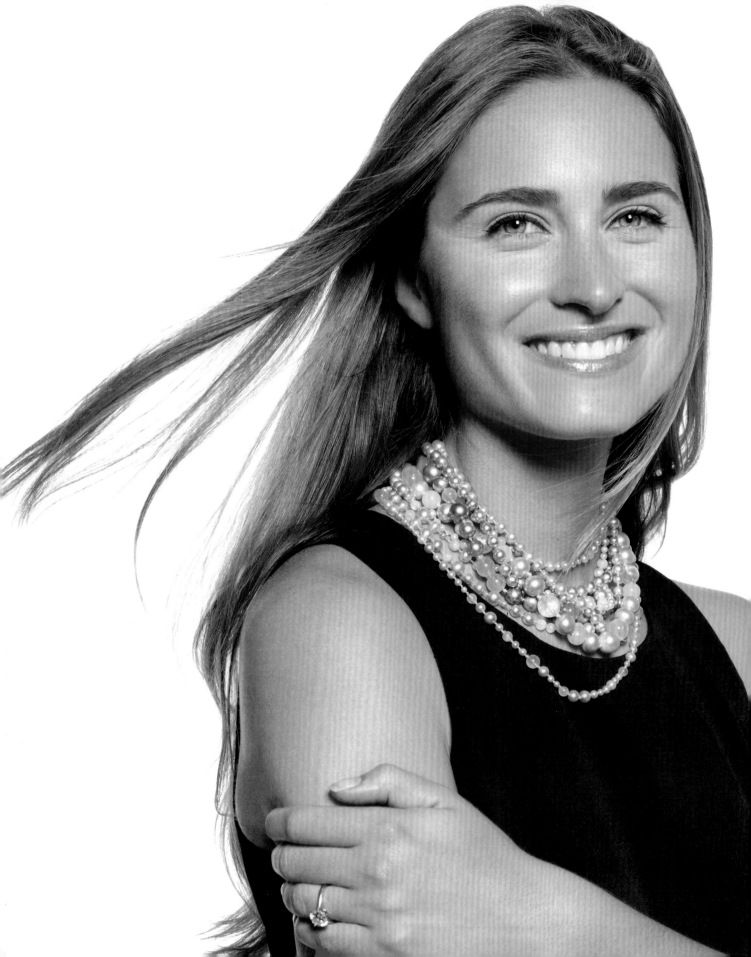

PRETTY NATURAL

Being Pretty Natural comes easily to women who are just that. It starts with a sparkle in the eye and amazingly clear skin. These women are the epitome of health and wellness and have the confidence and knowledge of what works for them. The women in this section are not only stunningly understated in their beauty, but they also understand that less is more and that subtle style simply works. I love women who are Pretty Natural because they know how to rock simplicity at its very best.

I am most comfortable when I am Pretty Natural. But it took me a while to get there. For years, I tried to emulate the blue-eyed blonde women who were on the covers of fashion magazines. When I arrived in the industry in NYC, I sat in the chairs of the top hairstylists and gave them free rein, but the results never looked like me. When it came to clothes, I even worked with major fashion stylists who brought me the latest looks, but I always felt as if I was wearing a costume. As for makeup, the natural evolution for me was about realizing that I looked best enhancing my coloring and sticking to who I am. I would love to be the very chic French woman who wears bright red lips or smoky eyes, but I'm not that person. I look and feel the most beautiful when I'm in subtle makeup, a simple outfit, and one or two pieces of amazing jewelry. That's all it takes. Simple, fresh, and modern is what works best for me. The bonus is how incredibly easy it is.

GETTING
THE NATURAL LOOK

A less-is-more approach to applying makeup

———

DAY

SKIN

You have healthy, clear skin that comes from eating right and taking care of yourself, so you want a foundation that looks completely natural, that you can't see on your skin. Begin with a dab of corrector and concealer just where you need it most, then a light foundation or tinted moisturizer that completely blends into skin.

CHEEKS

Go with a pretty blush that is the color your cheeks turn when you exercise.

EYES

If eyes are lined, it is very thin; anything dramatic would look out of place (and most days, mascara is enough). If you do use shadow, choose very subtle colors that work with the natural color of your eyelids.

LIPS

Choose a lip color in the natural tone that appears when you bite your lips (your perfect nude). You can achieve this by blotting regular lipstick, applying a pretty gloss, or reaching for a sheer lip stain.

HAIR

Pretty Natural hair should be healthy, shiny, carefree, and beautiful. A great cut that flatters the natural texture of the hair will give you an unfussy, low-maintenance look. Short cuts should flatter the shape of the face, while longer hair should be easy to maintain for wash-and-go chic.

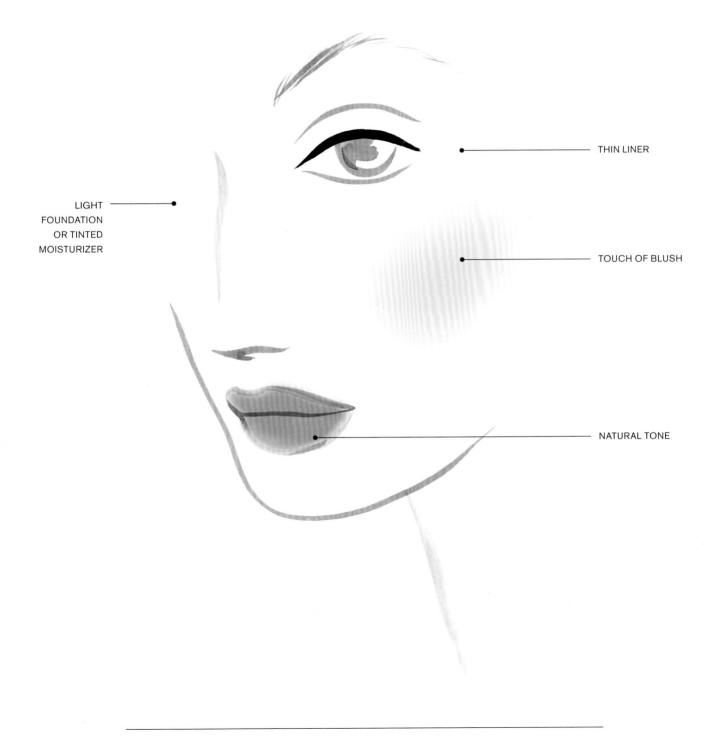

THIN LINER

LIGHT
FOUNDATION
OR TINTED
MOISTURIZER

TOUCH OF BLUSH

NATURAL TONE

GETTING
THE NATURAL LOOK

Just a touch of shimmer

EVENING

SKIN

For evening, you still want the weightless, invisible coverage that you use for day. Touching up your skin, with either a small amount of concealer or a few dabs of your daytime formula, is all you need for beautiful skin.

CHEEKS

On top of your daytime blush, add a bit of shimmer. Try a liquid or powder shimmer dabbed onto the top of the cheekbone for a subtle sparkle, or a clear balm over blush for some shine.

EYES

Play with texture in understated, natural colors like silver or champagne shimmer placed on the lid. If you don't usually line your eyes, try a thin black line on the upper lash line and an extra sweep of mascara.

LIPS

With natural makeup, a soft pale lip in a different texture than what you do for day—a gloss or shimmer—is a pretty choice. I also love the look of red lipstick and a fresh, bare face. It's simple and beautiful.

HAIR

A knot tied casually at the nape of the neck provides a carefree, unfussy party look for longer hair. With shorter styles, try adding a bit of product to keep the hair away from the face. This keeps the focus on your face and is a clean and modern way to style your hair.

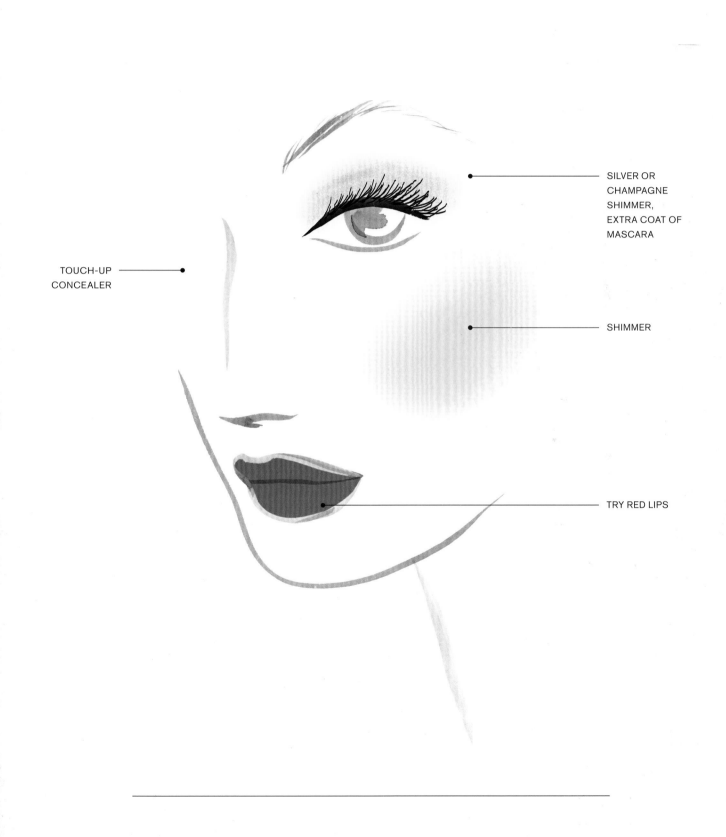

SILVER OR
CHAMPAGNE
SHIMMER,
EXTRA COAT OF
MASCARA

TOUCH-UP
CONCEALER

SHIMMER

TRY RED LIPS

ARE YOU
PRETTY NATURAL?

1
You love the healthy, natural glow that comes from wearing subtle makeup.

2
Your mantra is "Less is more."

3
When you're wearing dramatic makeup or a stylized haircut, you look at yourself and think, *Who is that woman?*

4
The secret to your fashion style is feeling comfortable. If you feel comfortable, you know that you look good in whatever you're wearing, even if it isn't the trend of the moment.

5
You feel most beautiful with a low-maintenance haircut that works with your natural texture.

6
You are a glass-half-full kind of person—you learned long ago that inner happiness and confidence radiate outwardly.

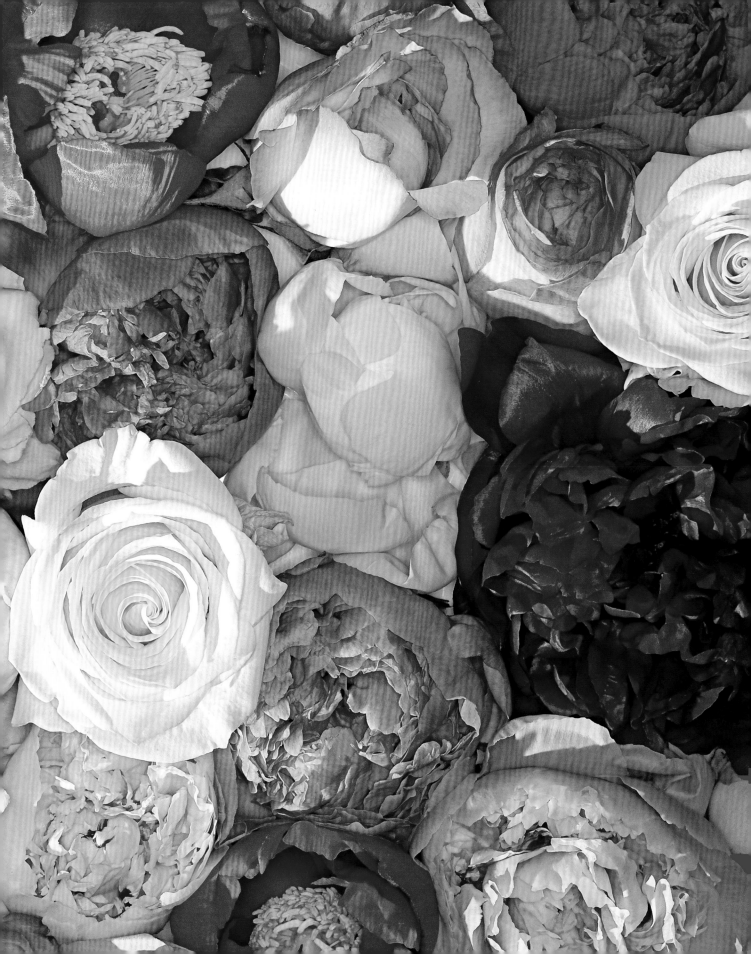

LAUREN BUSH
PHILANTHROPIST, MODEL, DESIGNER

———

Lauren Bush is a modern-day Grace Kelly, with glowing skin and perfect features. Lauren is very special; her eyes are full of light, and you can really see her kindness through them. She is naturally very giving and has done inspiring work with the FEED Foundation, which she cofounded. Through the UN World Food Programme, FEED has given more than sixty million school meals to children living in sixty-two of the poorest countries around the world.

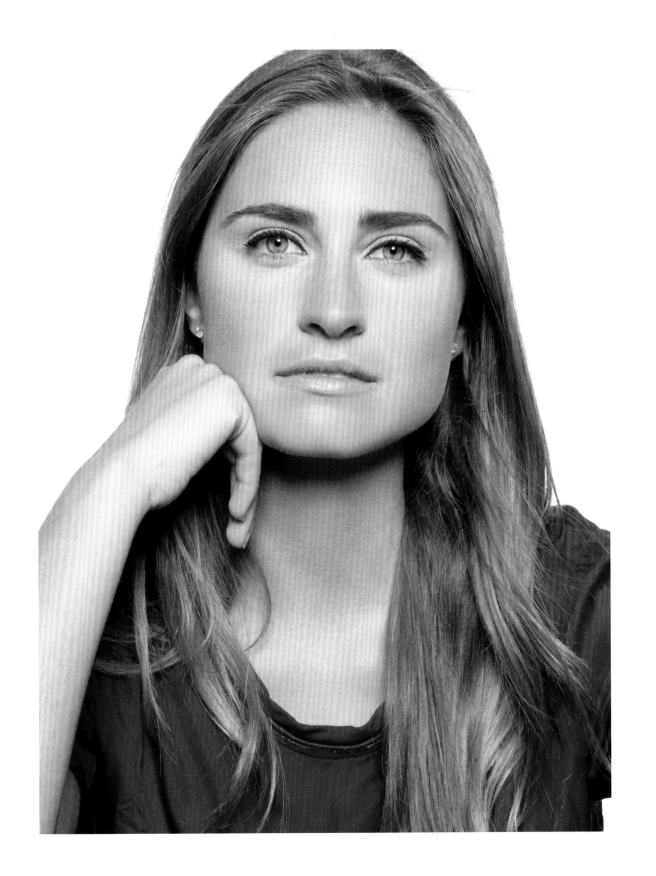

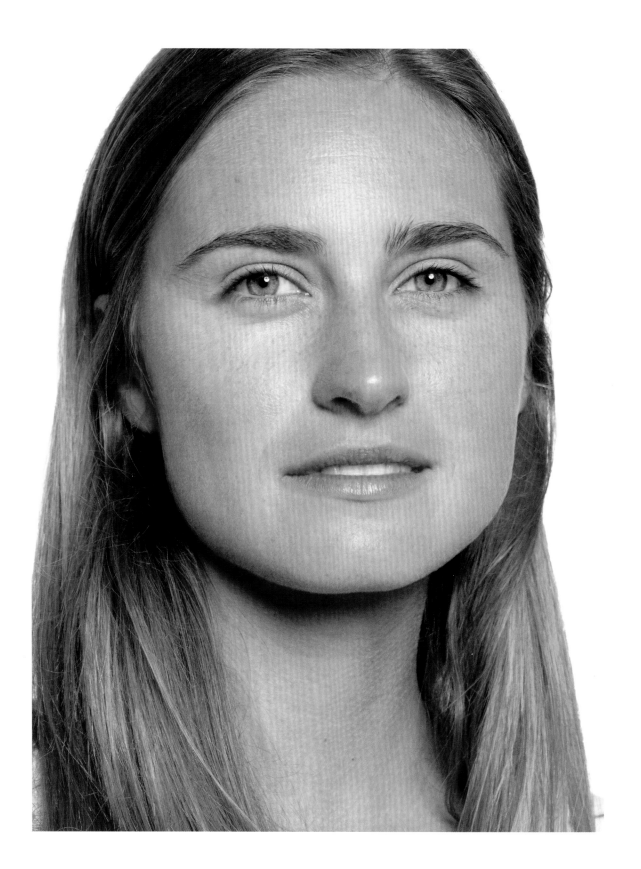

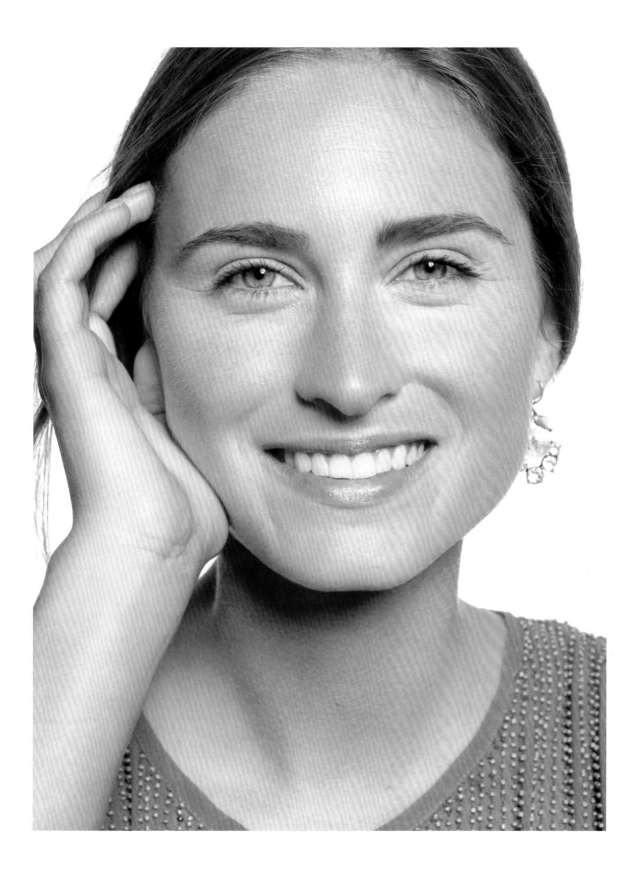

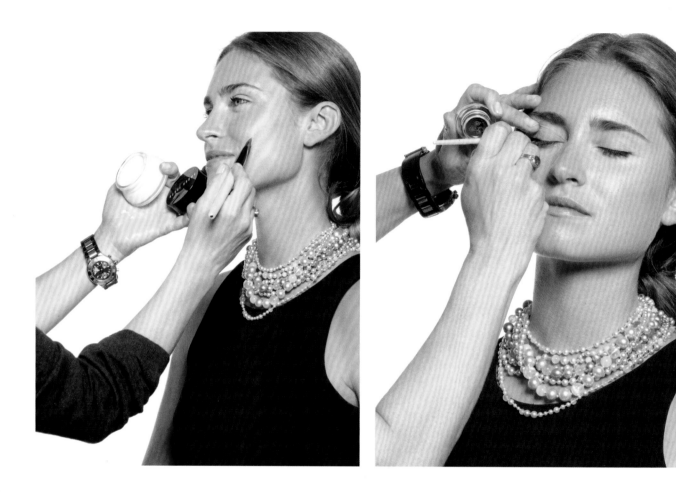

SKIN

Tinted moisturizer provides lightweight, almost sheer coverage and a gorgeous dewy finish. It is a great choice if you have great skin like Lauren. I like applying it with a brush because it deposits just the right amount.

EYES

To define Lauren's eyes, I drew a very thin line of black gel liner on the top lash line only. My trick for applying liner is to always start from the outer corner and draw the line inward. That way you ensure the most liner is deposited at the outer corner, avoiding clumps in the middle of the lash line. To ensure you have a smooth continuous line, open your eyes and fill in gaps where needed.

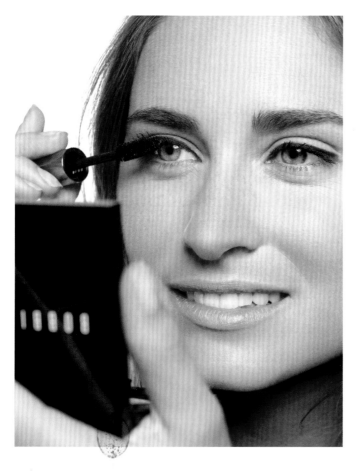

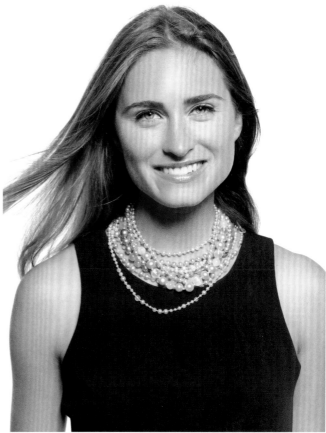

LASHES

The blacker the mascara, the better—it makes your eyes pop without having to put on a lot of eye shadow. Apply two to three coats underneath the top lashes, gently rolling the wand as you go to separate each lash.

THE LOOK

Sandy pink blush on the apples of Lauren's cheeks and a sheer pink gloss complete Lauren's easy natural look. For added glow, pearls always bring light to the face.

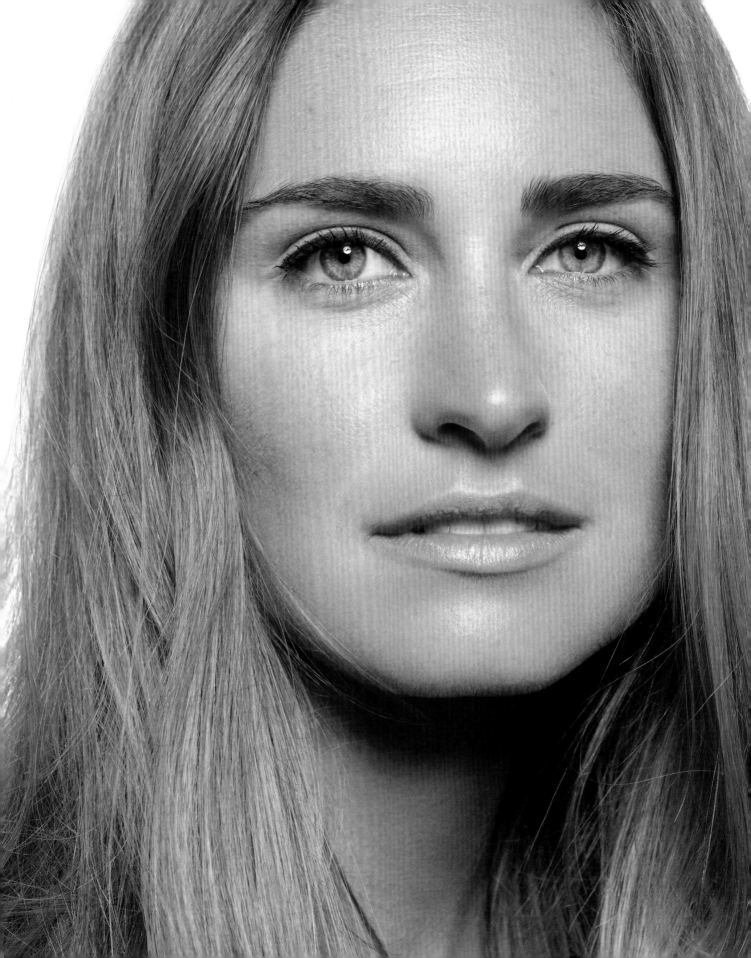

Treat others the way you would want to be treated.

—LAUREN BUSH

The best advice I ever received was to just get started. The hardest part is when you have a great idea but it is only in your head. So just to believe in yourself—putting one foot in front of the other and getting the wheels in motion—is the only way you will know if your idea is going to work or not. You will never know unless you start.

The biggest challenge I've overcome so far is self-doubt. So many of us face this, and it can be crippling at times. We waste so much time doubting ourselves—I did for four years during middle school. It just paralyzes you from realizing your true potential. I feel really grateful to have come out of that and come into my own doing something that I love.

I was a very sensitive person growing up, but now I feel like that led me to what I'm doing now. I think if I weren't so sensitive, I wouldn't be who I am, so I've learned to embrace it.

Treat others the way you would want to be treated. I guess it is corny, but I think if everyone lived by that, the world would really be a better place.

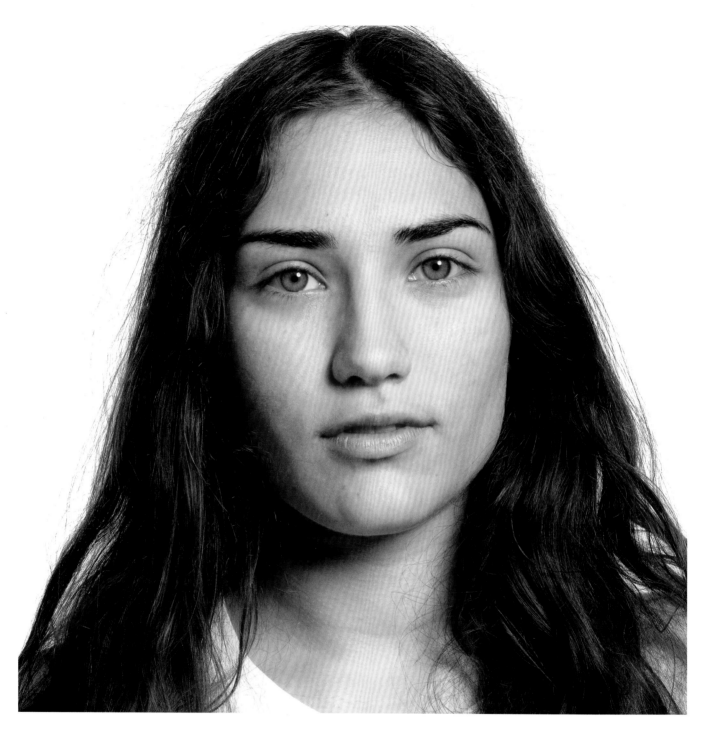

ABBY STEDMAN PRODUCTION ASSISTANT

A pot of peppermint tea is what makes me feel beautiful on a bad day.

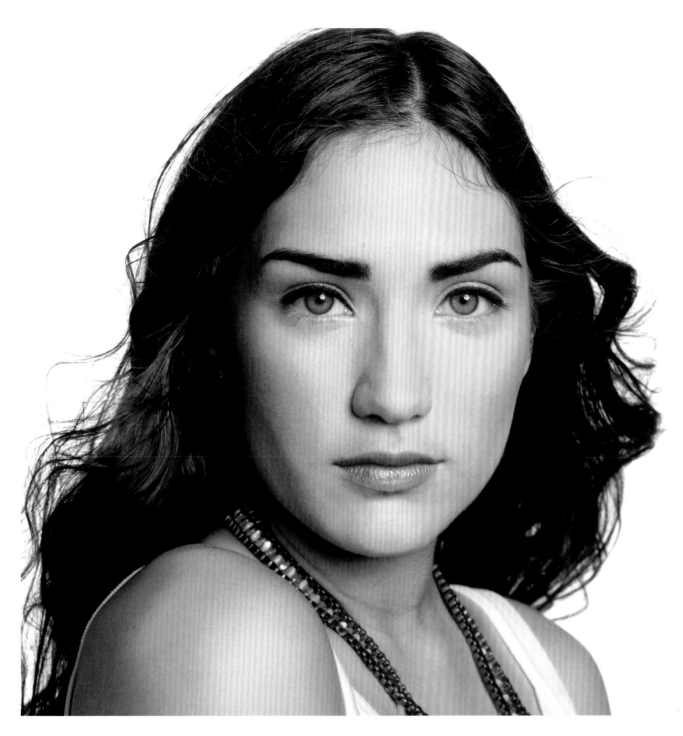

ABBY'S MAKEUP

When you have striking brows like Abby, you should enhance their beautiful color and shape. On Abby, we filled in and defined her brows with a slanted hard-edged eyebrow brush and a rich mahogany shadow that matches her hair color. To open up and highlight Abby's sparkling green eyes, we used a gel liner in the same rich brown shade and applied a pale shimmery green cream shadow from the lash line up to the crease. Soft pink cheeks and pinky lips with a touch of shimmer complete her easy, gorgeous evening look.

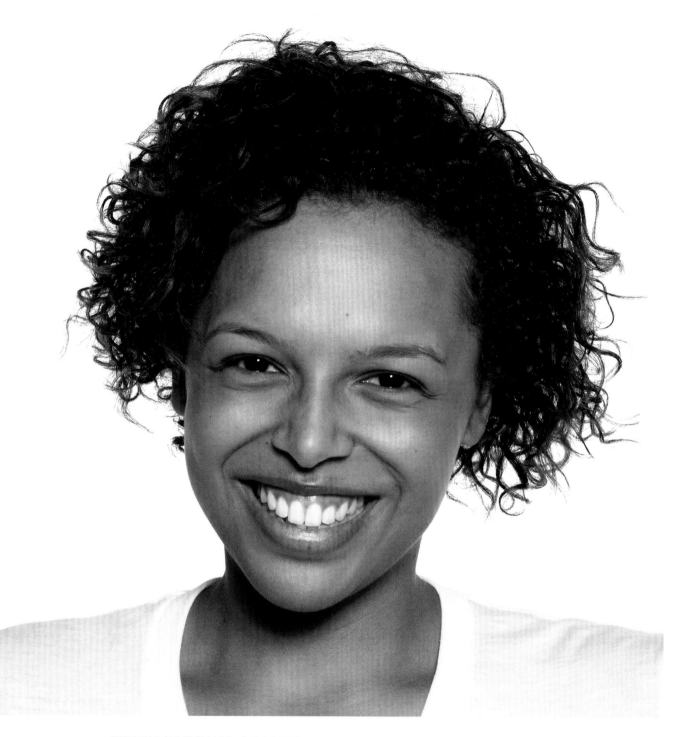

KIRBY BUMPUS GRANTS MANAGER, POVERTY FIGHTER

*It's taken some time, but I finally started loving my hair in college when
I realized it looks cute naturally curly, blown out, and in braids.*

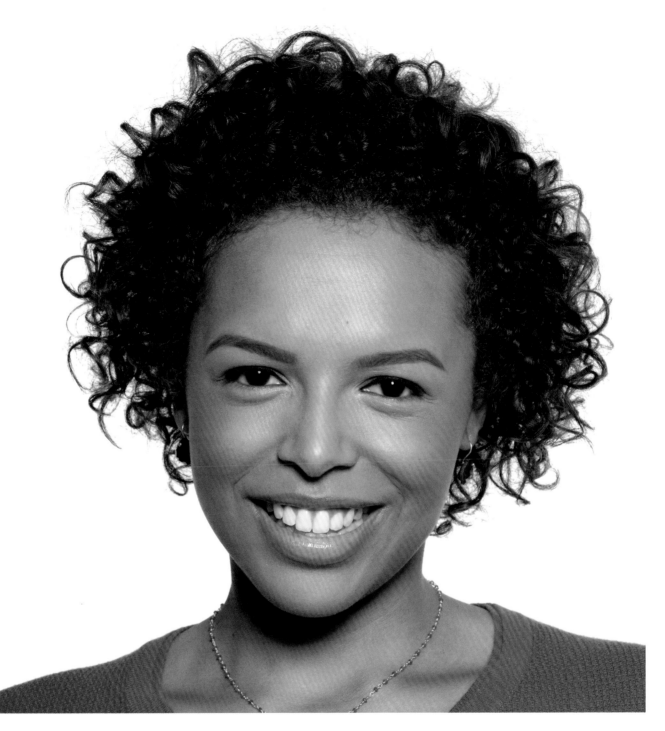

KIRBY'S MAKEUP

To draw attention to a great smile, you don't necessarily need a bold lip color—sometimes soft and pale is better. A sweet pink lipstick topped with a pink gloss lets Kirby shine.

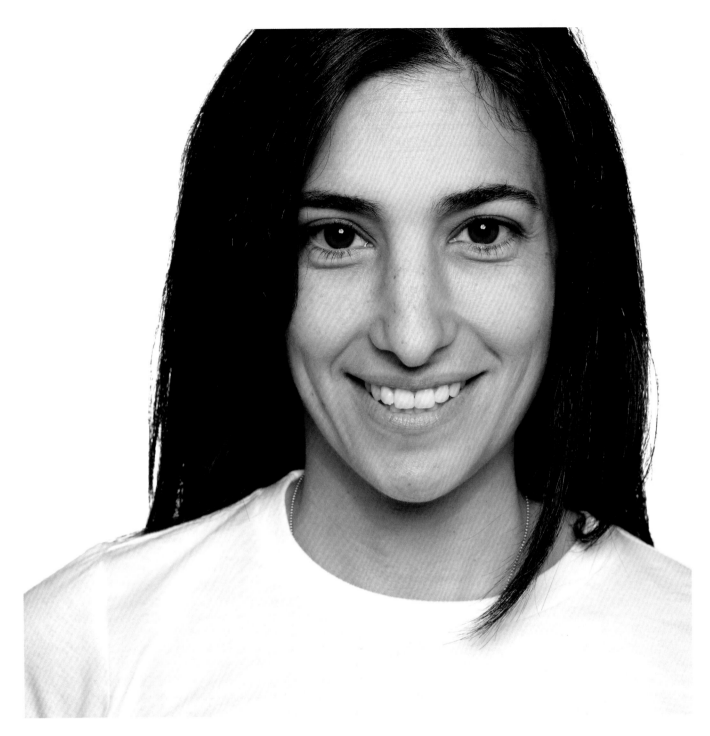

GABRIELLE NEVIN PRODUCT DEVELOPMENT

*I like the rich brown color of my eyes and hair. Funny because growing
up, all I wanted was blonde hair and blue eyes!*

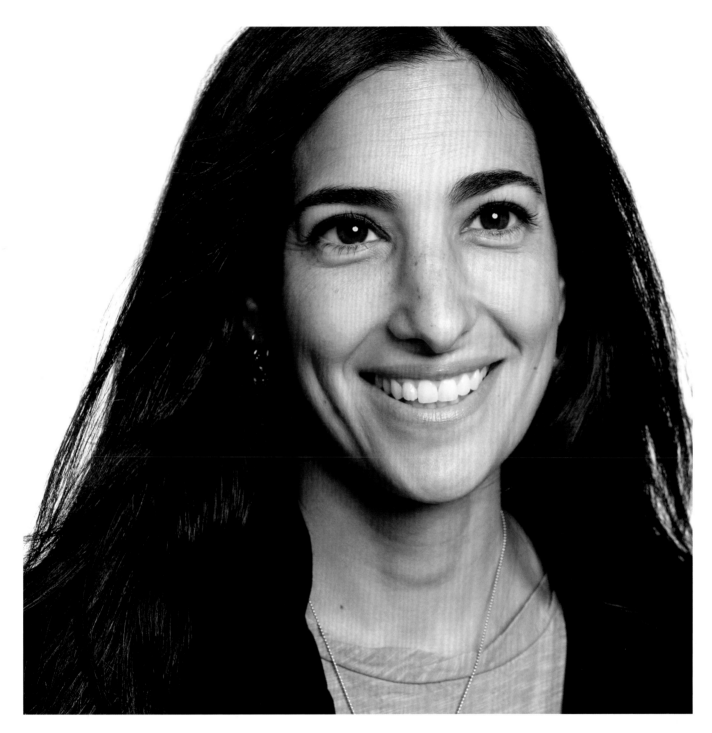

GABRIELLE'S MAKEUP

I truly believe less is more, and Gabby is a perfect example of how minimal makeup is often all you need for a vibrant, gorgeous look. We added a little concealer and foundation where needed. To give her brows a little polish, we brushed them up with a clear gel. Then we applied dark brown gel liner and two coats of black mascara. Sandy pink blush really wakes up her complexion. Because Gabby's lips are already a lovely shade of pink, we chose a pretty neutral pinky-nude lip color that enhances her natural shade.

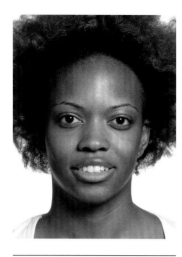

APRIL PERRY
BARTENDER,
ASPIRING SINGER,
ACTRESS

The best compliment I've ever received is that I bring sunshine into the room.

APRIL'S MAKEUP

Many women think bronzer is just for looking tan, but I use it for blending, correcting, and adding warmth. After evening out April's skin with a foundation stick using a brush, we relied on a warm bronzer and coral shimmer blush on her cheeks to give her a warm lit-from-within glow. For April's eyes, we began with a bone eye shadow base and bronze metallic shimmer eye shadow on the lid that echoes the same warm tones we used on her skin. An apricot pot rouge applied with a brush and topped with a clear gloss adds a cheerful touch of color to her lips.

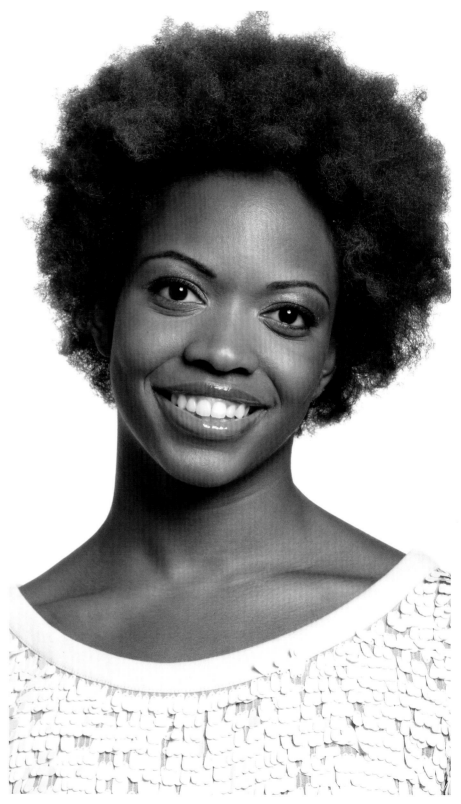

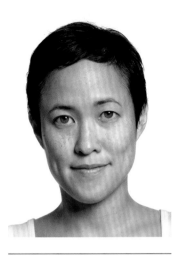

MARIE CLARE KATIGBAK
COPYWRITER

Now that I'm in my thirties, undereye concealer is an every-day essential. It makes me look fresh and bright-eyed, even when I'm not.

MARIE CLARE'S MAKEUP

When you have beautiful skin like Marie Clare, great skincare, rather than foundation, is all you need for an even-toned, glowing complexion. For instant radiance, we relied on brightening serum followed by brightening moistur-izer. These are formulas that not only moisturize, but also, over time, help skin become clearer and more radiant. To even out dark patches, we used a spot corrector that matched her skin tone. Pale pink blush adds a touch of color, while a sheer metallic shadow with a hint of green brings out her stun-ning green eyes. High-shine clear lip gloss completes her gorgeous low-maintenance look.

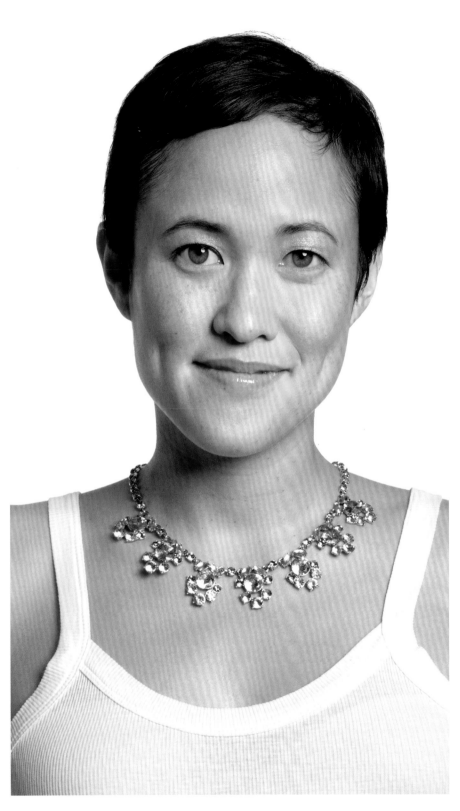

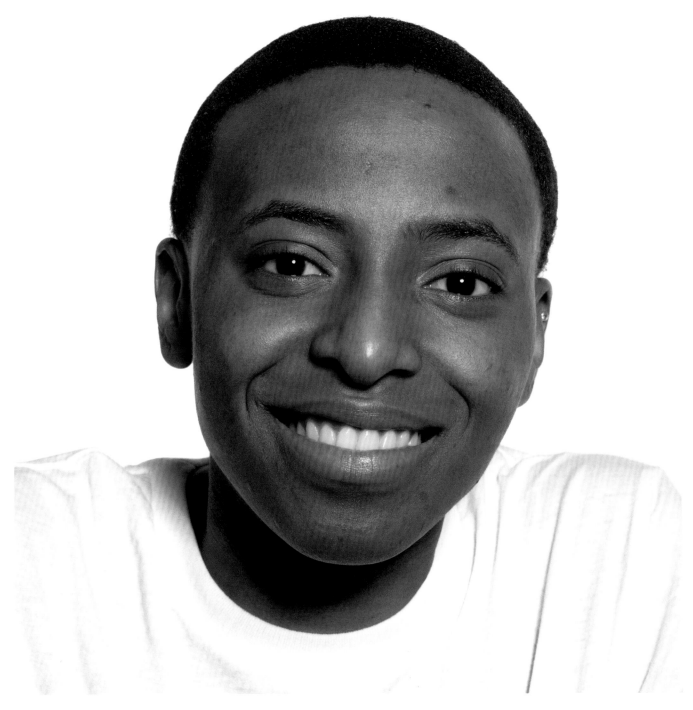

JAY GOLSON ASPIRING FASHION STYLIST

The best beauty advice I've received is to stay true to yourself—I always have and I always will.

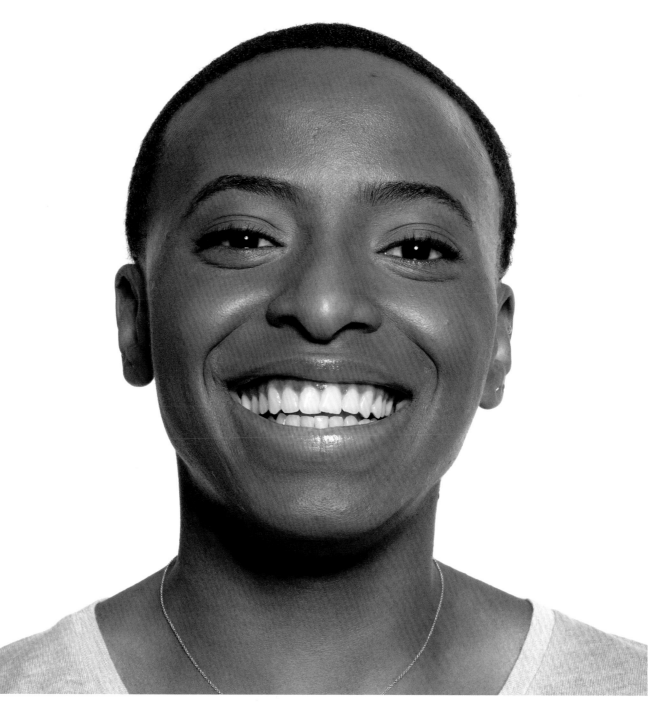

JAY'S MAKEUP

It was so much fun to do Jay's face because she had never worn makeup a day in her life! Some tinted moisturizer and a shimmer blush brought out her luminescence. To play up Jay's gorgeous brown eyes, I applied a toast shadow all over the lid as a base and then added depth with a richer cocoa shade on the lower part of the lid. A sweep of soft charcoal shadow for the liner and few coats of mascara was all it took to make Jay's eyes pop.

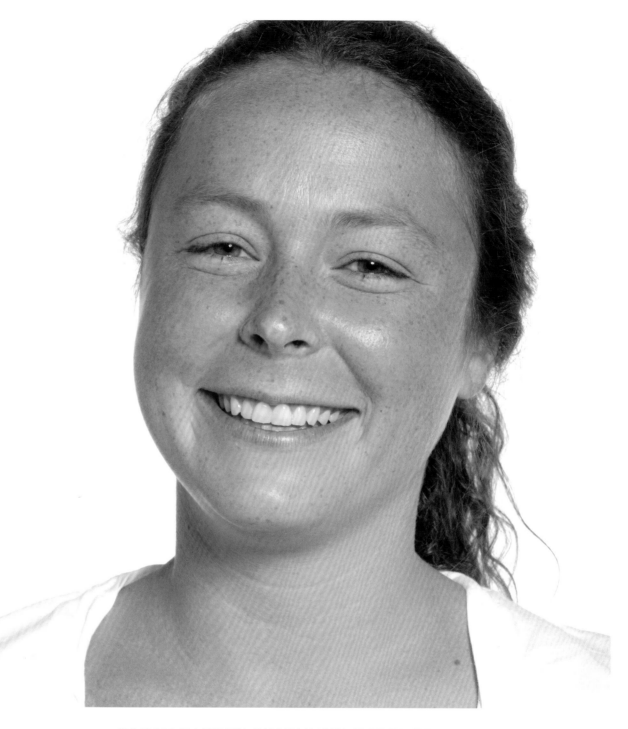

SARAH CARDEN SUSTAINABLE FARMER

I'm happiest after a hard day. Conquering challenging days makes me feel incredibly rewarded and satisfied. That feeling of hard-earned fatigue creates a lot of satisfaction in me.

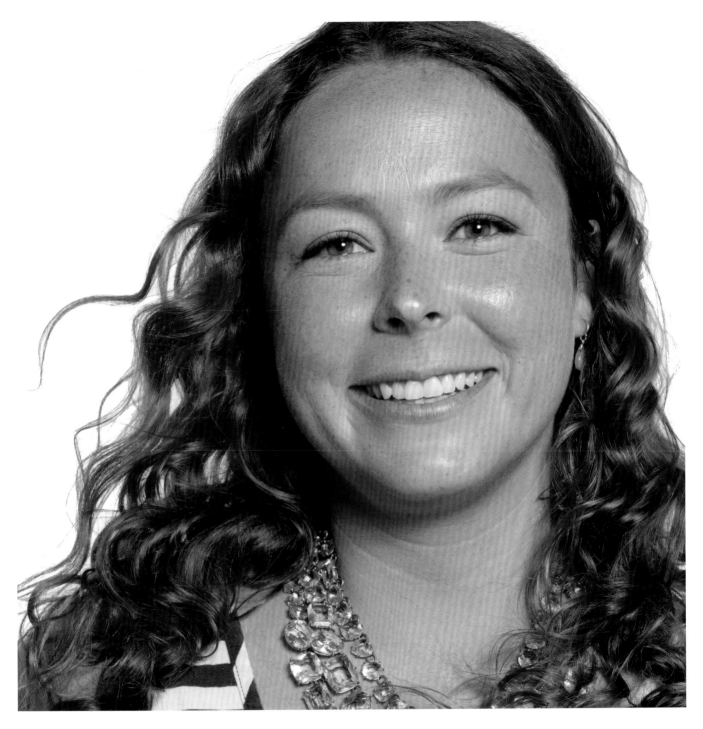

SARAH'S MAKEUP

To celebrate Sarah's fresh, outdoorsy glow and natural sparkle, we kept her makeup to a minimum. When you spend a lot of time outside like Sarah, it's common to have some redness. We toned hers down with tinted moisturizer and a yellow-based loose powder. Her lips have plenty of natural color, so we kept them bare and enhanced her smile with bronzer topped with dusty pink powder blush.

CINDI LEIVE
EDITOR IN CHIEF OF *GLAMOUR* MAGAZINE

———

As the editor in chief of *Glamour*, Cindi provides answers and inspiration for smart women, encouraging them to be their best selves. Cindi is down-to-earth and real, despite having a very high-profile, high-powered career. Her warm and positive personality is reflected in her easy style. Even when she is wearing a designer dress during Fashion Week, she is still beautifully understated.

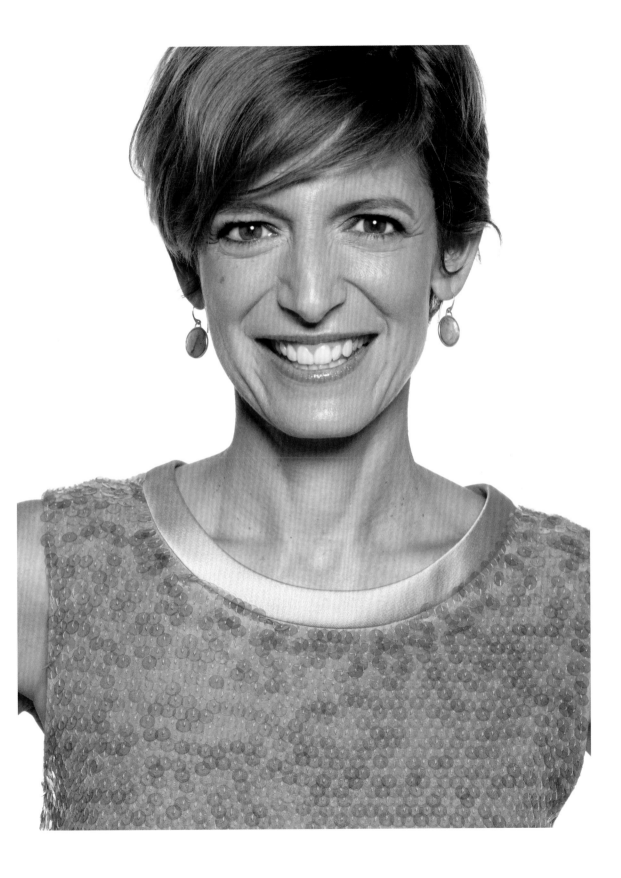

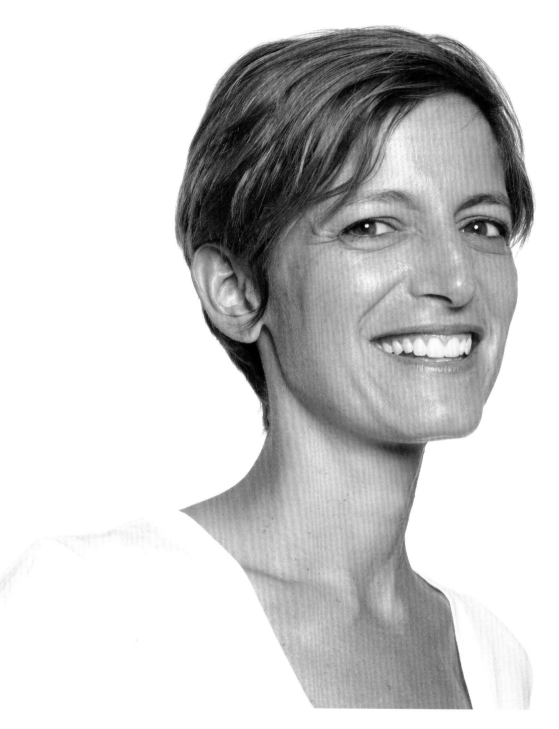

CINDI WITHOUT MAKEUP

Cindi has a brilliant mind and positive energy to spare. I have always told Cindi how much I love her look.
She rocks her short hair, and her nose is adorable and one of her best features.

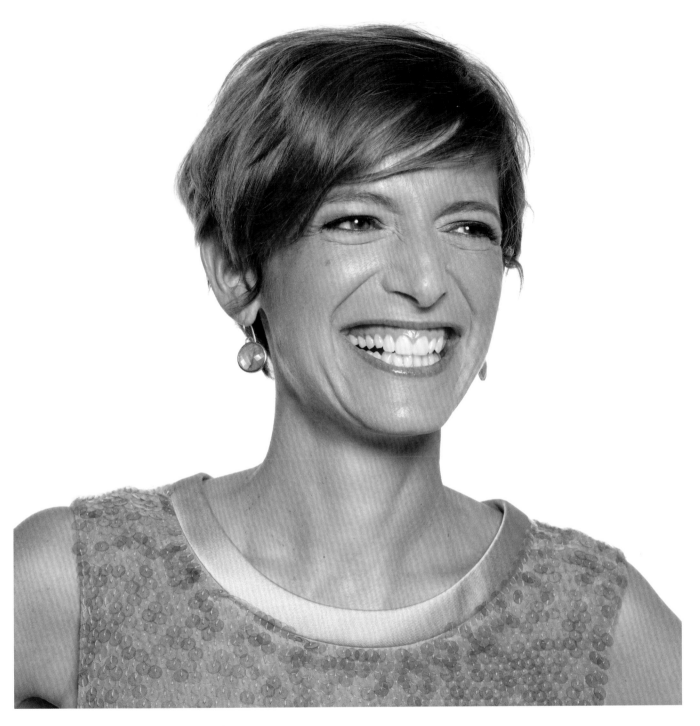

CINDI WITH MAKEUP

When you have beautiful skin like Cindi, you don't want to cover it up with heavy makeup. A tinted moisturizer is a great option for sheer, natural-looking coverage. For Cindi's eyes, I gave her a softer, more natural version of a smoky eye by layering a chocolate shadow liner on top of black gel liner—it is a trick that makes her eyes stand out without being overpowering. To give Cindi some added sparkle that works for day as well as night, I layered a creamy pink blush with a bit of shimmer on top.

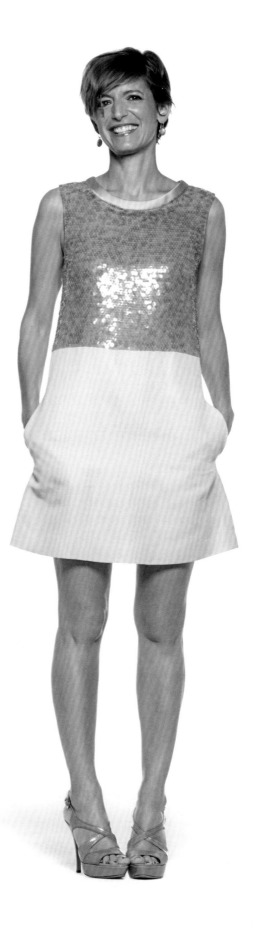

Something that seems like an obstacle usually isn't.

—CINDI LEIVE

I love my short hair because it's easy. It was such a revelation to me that I could have hair that took exactly three and a half minutes to dry in the morning.

I have never been a foundation person, because I hate that feeling of wearing a mask. Discovering tinted moisturizer was a very good thing.

Now I see my nose as something that makes me look like me, but in seventh grade I was incredibly insecure about it. The bump in my nose was all I could think about thanks to friends (or frenemies) commenting on it. But of course, these are things that you have to go through to get to that ultimate place where you feel good about your looks.

Something that seems like an obstacle usually isn't. I had a boss who always said, "When one door closes, another one opens." While it sounds like a cliché, it really is true, and I find it such a reassuring thing to know.

I was super driven and pretty independent when I was in college. So I think if I could give advice to my eighteen-year-old self, I would tell myself to slow down, put your feet up, and enjoy a margarita.

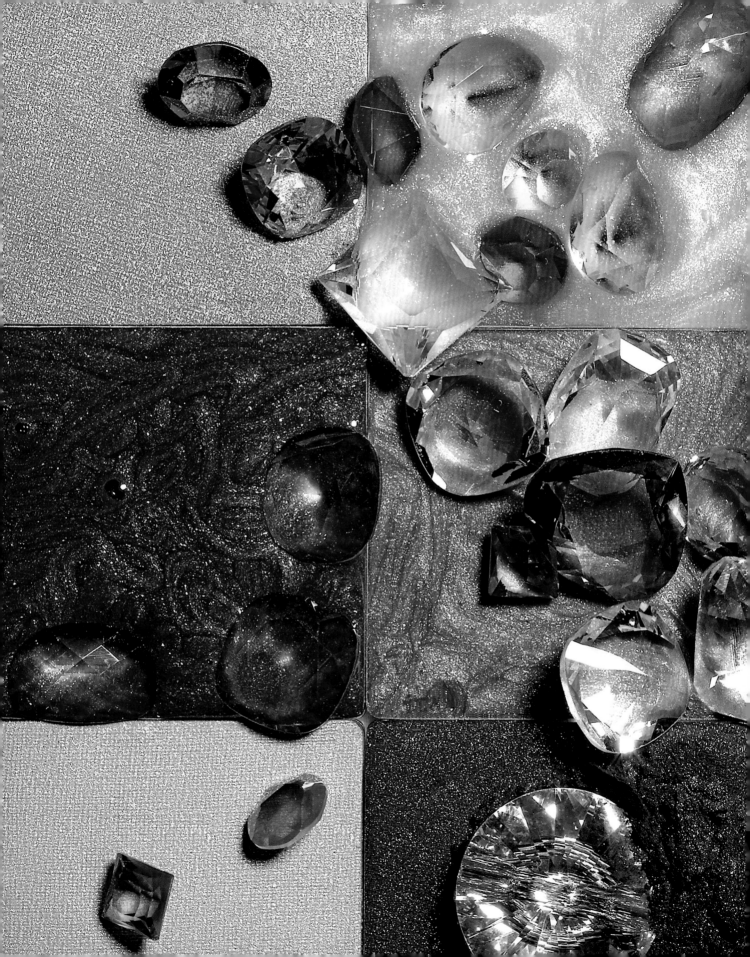

02

PRETTY RADIANT

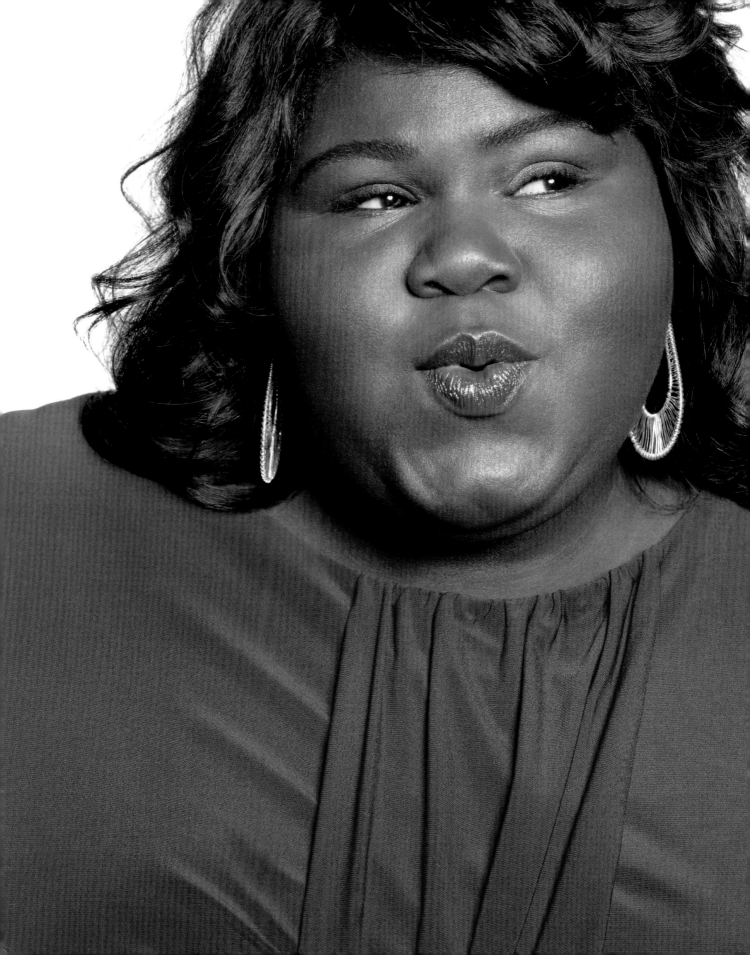

PRETTY RADIANT

Women who are Pretty Radiant instantly light up a room with their positive energy. Radiance isn't only something you see, but you feel it immediately. These dynamic women have the natural ability to make people laugh, open up, and relax—without even trying. Michelle Obama is a Pretty Radiant woman—she walks into a room and brings it to life. Women who are radiant are happy at their core. They eat well and exercise, and they don't hold on to negative thoughts.

Pretty Radiant women use both beauty and style to express their personalities. This doesn't mean over-the-top, look-at-me makeup or clothing—they get noticed even when they are simply dressed. It's more about expressing their individuality with just a pop of color or a touch of sparkle. It's a purple trench on a rainy day, a pair of gold pumps, or rhinestone jewelry. They choose pieces that make their look come alive. I like to be Pretty Radiant when it comes to my own makeup—especially at night. With makeup, I focus on bringing light and sparkle to my face with a touch of shimmer to the cheekbones and a pretty hue of creamy pot rouge on both lips and cheeks. I play up my eyes with a sweep of liner and a glimmer of color (and tons of mascara). I love being with women who are Pretty Radiant because they shine, and they are the people you want around all the time.

GETTING THE GLOW

Beauty tips for looking absolutely radiant

———

DAY

SKIN

Start with completely clean skin, then layer on moisturizers that are right for your skin type until you can actually see the hydration and glow. You want your face to be not only hydrated, but also smooth and almost creamy. For a dewier look, pat a bit of face oil onto cheeks.

After adding corrector and concealer where needed, even out your skin with a color-correct foundation (or a rich tinted moisturizer for natural coverage). The trick is having your skin look plump and moisturized but not greasy. Blend away any extra shine with a sponge or your fingers.

CHEEKS

To bring color, warmth, and sheen to your face, apply a creamy blush or pot rouge. Shimmer powder looks gorgeous when dusted on cheekbones. Just make sure it doesn't mix with moisturizer, or it can crease.

EYES

Eyeliner and mascara are a simple way to bring definition to your eyes. Adding sheer gloss to your lids makes them shine. Light-reflective shimmer shadows are a beautiful way to add sparkle.

LIPS

Add creamy lipstick in a shade that's pretty and not too strong. There is a rose hue for everyone. If you have color in your lips naturally, just apply gloss.

HAIR

Pretty Radiant hair should be a beautiful shape to frame your face and keep the spotlight on your smile. Work with your natural texture, using products that keep it healthy and shiny. Highlights in varying shades add light and luminosity to your face.

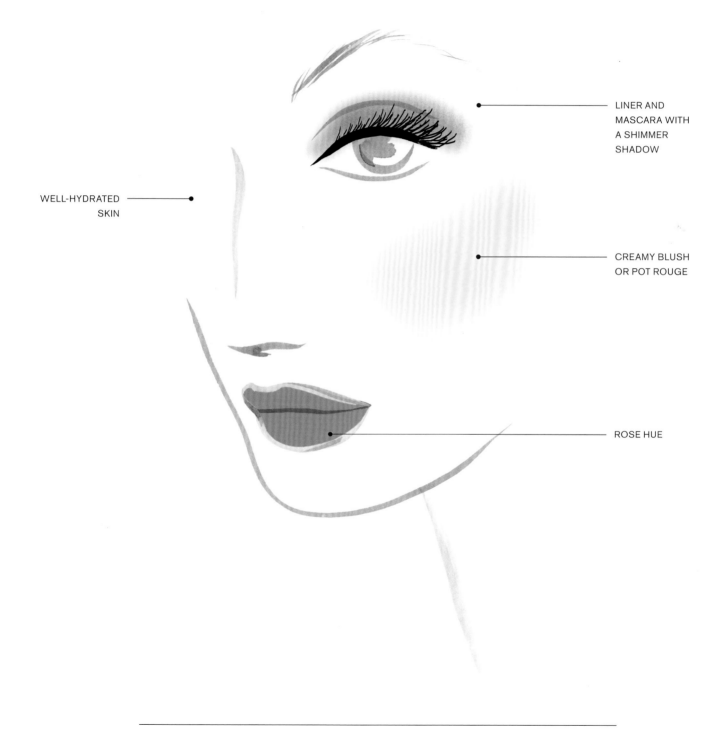

LINER AND
MASCARA WITH
A SHIMMER
SHADOW

WELL-HYDRATED
SKIN

CREAMY BLUSH
OR POT ROUGE

ROSE HUE

GETTING THE GLOW

Turn up the color

—

EVENING

SKIN

You still want to have glowing skin for night, but you'll want a little more coverage. If you use a tinted moisturizing balm during the day, at night try switching to a light- to medium-coverage foundation for a more polished finish.

CHEEKS

To add radiance to your face, try a pop of something brighter or bolder. Stick with the same formulas you use for day but amp up the color. A brighter pink for fair skin, or cranberry or plum for darker skin, gives you an extra glow.

EYES

For women with darker skin, go with gold and burnished colors and a thicker line of black liner. For women with fairer skin, experiment with a smokier eye than usual, adding a bit more depth with a skin tone shimmer on the lower lid and a darker shade in the crease. Bump up the mascara with an extra coat or two.

LIPS

Add a little more power to your lips with a formula one shade stronger for night. For a modern, luminous lip, try a red gloss.

HAIR

A subtle yet still feminine change for night works best for Pretty Radiant women. Try finger waves for soft cascading curls, get an elegant blowout, or put your hair up in a beautiful upsweep.

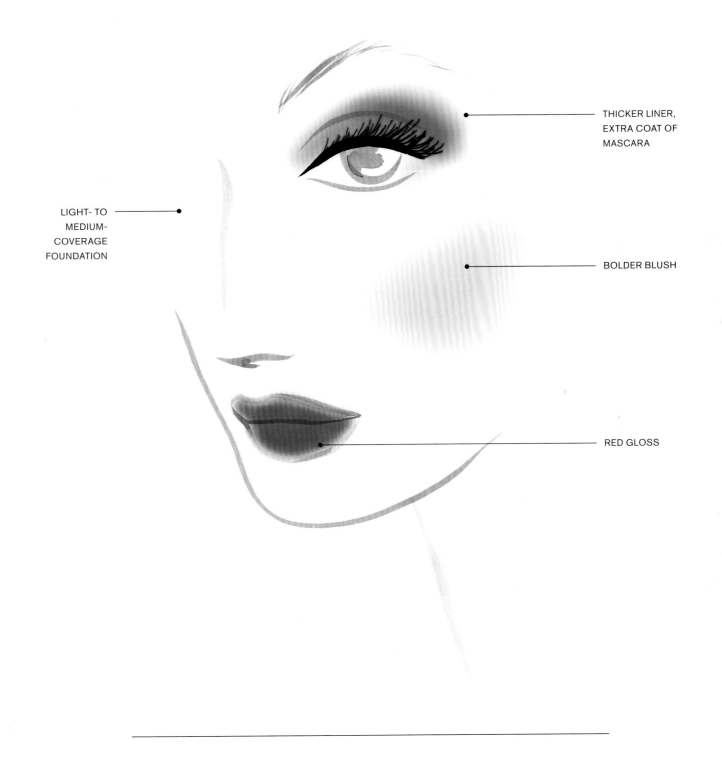

THICKER LINER,
EXTRA COAT OF
MASCARA

LIGHT- TO
MEDIUM-
COVERAGE
FOUNDATION

BOLDER BLUSH

RED GLOSS

GABOUREY SIDIBE
ACTRESS

———

I first met Gabby when she was nominated for a Golden Globe for *Precious*, and I did her makeup for the event. She was a brand-new star who was suddenly lighting up the covers of major magazines. Gabby was so open and humble and excited about the process of becoming famous. She had this "Wow!" sense about her. Gabby works with my team all the time, and we've gotten to know her well. She is super funny with a really smart wit. She's constantly giggling and cracking everyone up. What I love most about Gabby is that she's really comfortable in her own skin. She's happy to be who she is.

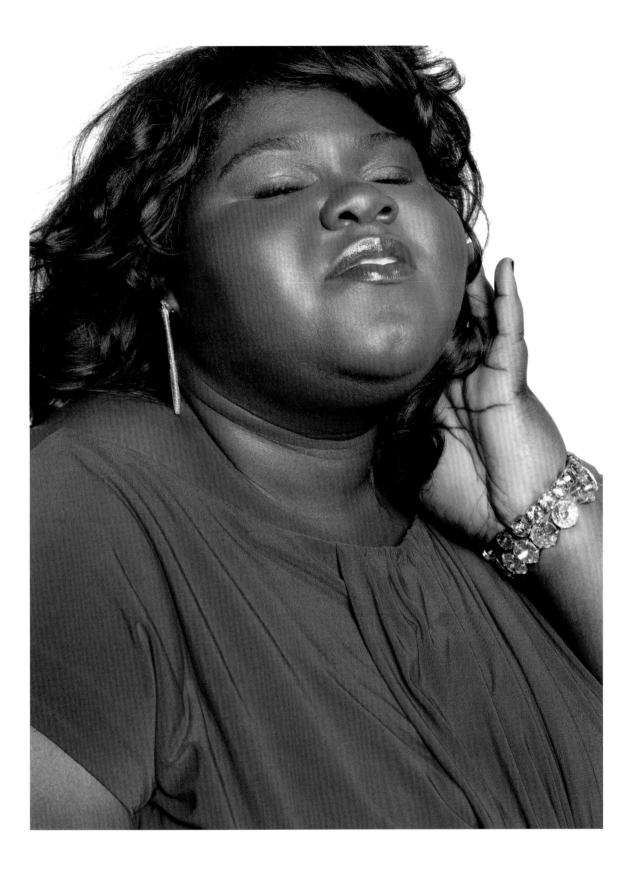

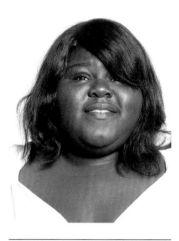

GABOUREY WITHOUT MAKEUP

Gabby is one of those people who smiles with her eyes—it's beautiful. And she's lucky to have skin that is luminescent. Two minutes of makeup is all she needs.

GABOUREY'S MAKEUP

Currant-colored blush with a natural chocolate lip color instantly wakes up Gabby's face. Black eyeliner and lengthening mascara, along with a clear gel brushed on the brows, open up her eyes and give Gabby a polished, pretty look.

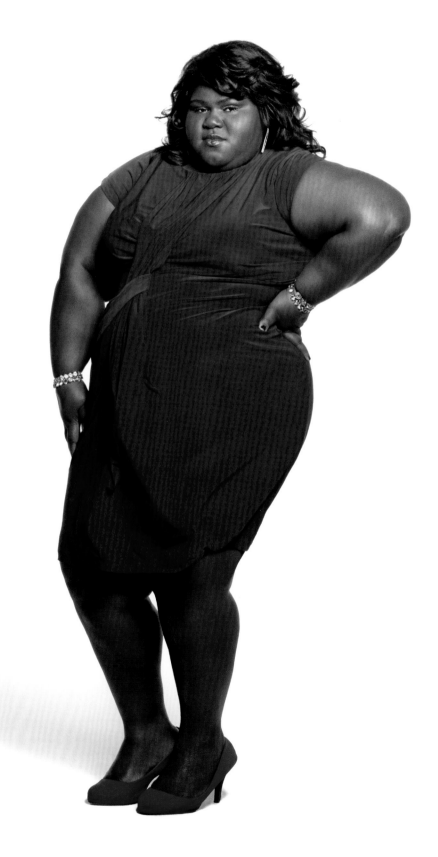

A lot of my power comes from sheer will and confidence.

—GABOUREY SIDIBE

I think there is a silver lining in everything. I don't believe in regret. I only believe in situations that you can learn from.

I've had to overcome what people think of me. People have misconceptions about people who are bigger, or darker, or younger, and everything that I happen to be. So no matter what they are thinking at that time, I have to get over it and be who I am despite what they think.

I consider myself a powerful woman just because I know who I am. I know what my likes and dislikes are, and that is a huge part of finding your own power.

I'm happiest when I am in my room putting on makeup, trying on different colors for no particular reason. Not because I have someplace to go, but just because I like to play.

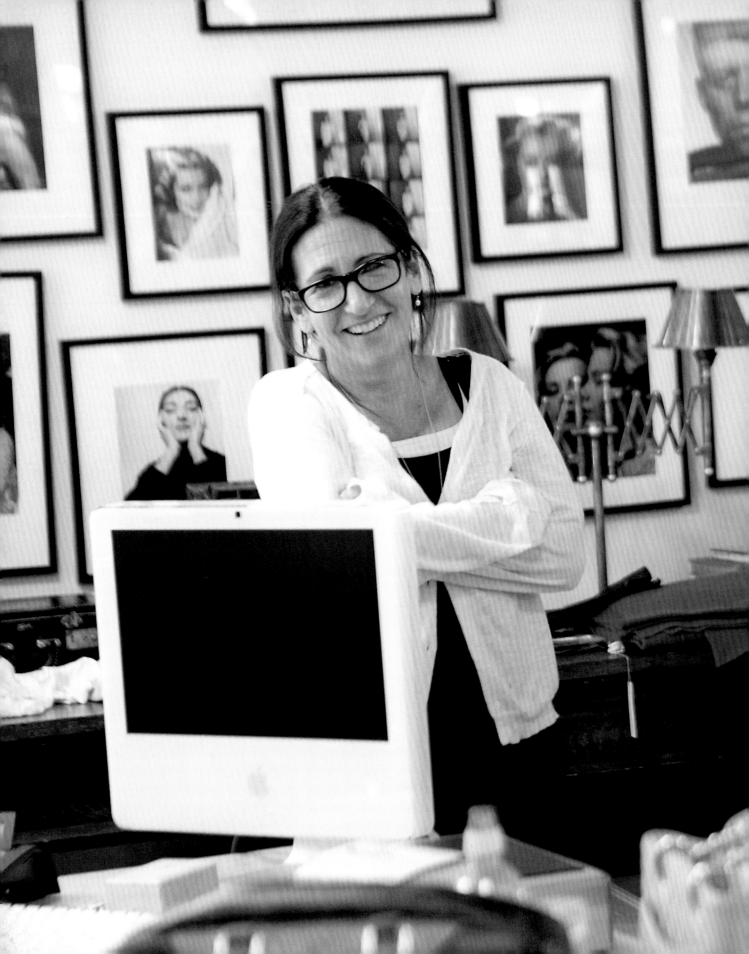

DOING WHAT
YOU LOVE

I am fortunate to be passionate about what I do. Makeup, color, and everything visual have always been what makes me happy. Thanks to my parents, who understood the importance of pursuing my passion, I made makeup my major in college—a first at my school. I knew that I would eventually turn my fascination with makeup, and how it can transform women inside and out, into a career.

When you do what you love, it doesn't feel like work. This doesn't mean there won't be challenging or exhausting days, but if you really enjoy something, that helps carry you through the inevitable tough parts. Maybe it is your full-time job or what you do when you clock out, but whether you are a mother, a volunteer, a CEO, or an artist, finding the things that make you light up is what life is all about.

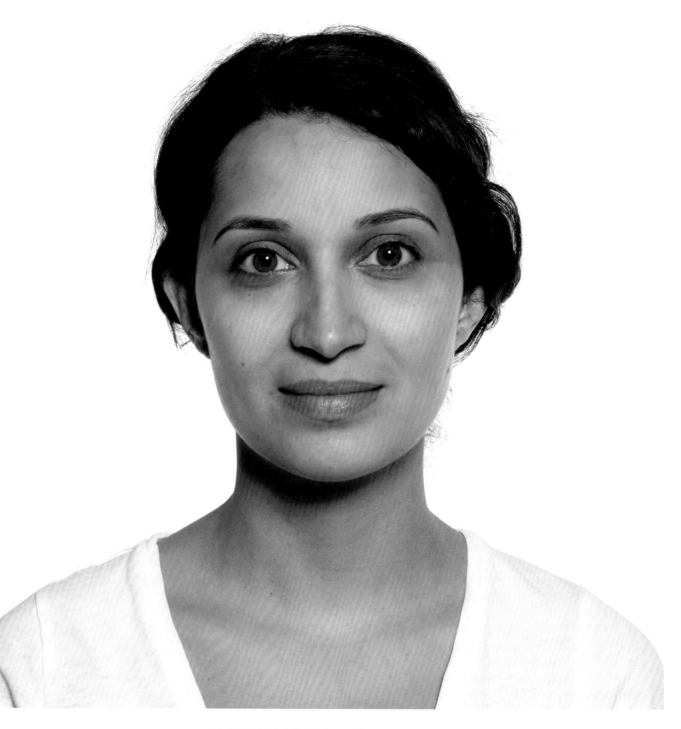

ALEXIS RODRIGUEZ PUBLICIST

The person I admire most is my mother. She has overcome so much adversity in her life. My morals, work ethic, perseverance, confidence, and strength are all a result of the incredible role model that is my mother.

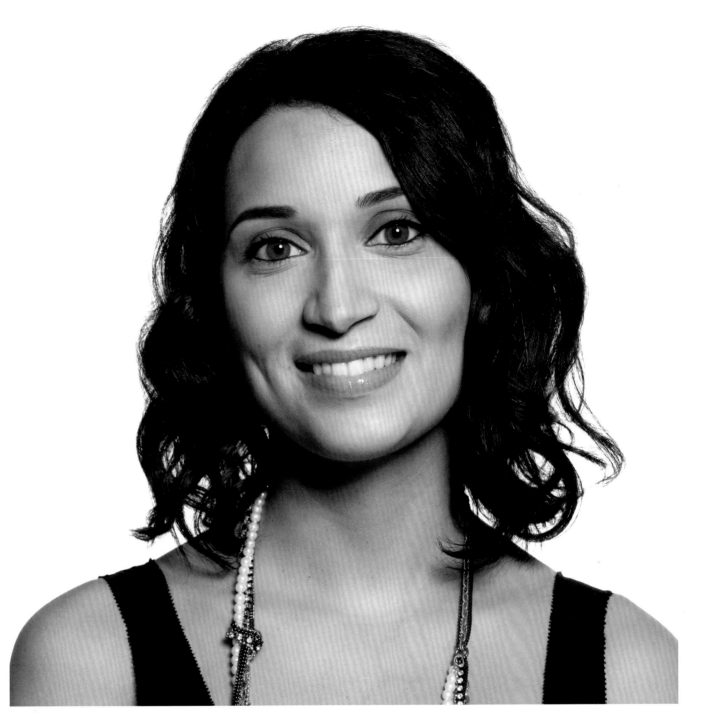

ALEXIS'S MAKEUP

If you are lucky enough to have a pretty natural shadow on your lids like Alexis, you don't need a lot of eye shadow. I just added a bit of sheen on the lids. Underneath the eyes, I neutralized any darkness with a corrector and then used a concealer to add brightness. Black gel liner on the top lash line, and a black pencil on the inner lower lash plus several coats of black mascara, brought even more depth to her stunning eyes. Alexis has a great natural lip color, so all she needed was a touch of gloss to finish the look.

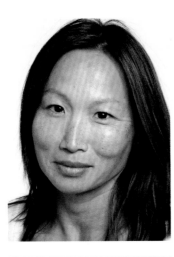

LEE HEH MARGOLIES
HOUSEHOLD CEO

If I focus on my beauty flaws, it becomes a downward spiral, so I have learned as I've gotten older to not even go there! I prefer to focus on confidence and comfort. Hopefully that gets projected as outward beauty.

LEE HEH'S MAKEUP

I love the look of Lee Heh's freckles and smile. To even out her skin while allowing her freckles to shine through, we spot-applied a foundation stick with a foundation brush only where skin was uneven. To define brows that were lighter than her hair, we relied on a dark brown brow pencil in the same shade as Lee Heh's hair. To further bring out her eyes, we drew a thick line of black powder eye shadow along the top lash line and dusted a shimmery champagne shadow on her lids.

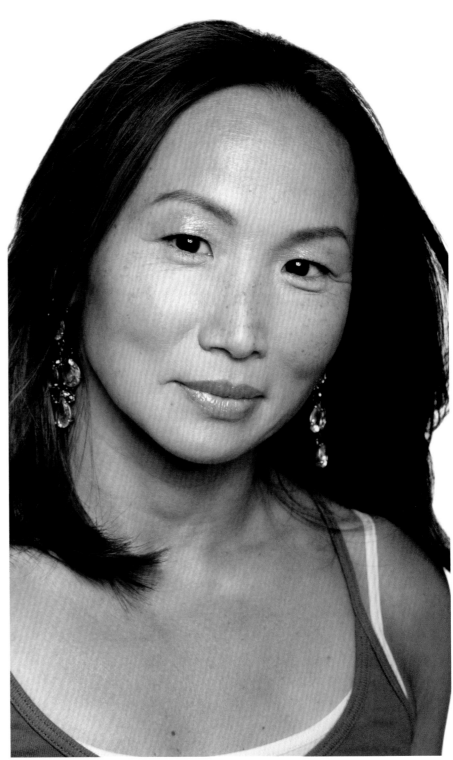

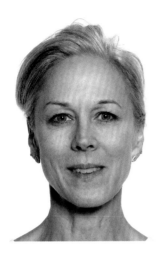

GRO FRIVOLL
SVP GLOBAL
CREATIVE
DIRECTOR

I see my face as a blank canvas, so when I'm getting ready in the morning, every stroke of blush, eye shadow, mascara, and lipstick brings it to life. I find the transformation to be a very cathartic experience.

GRO'S MAKEUP

To make Gro's eyebrows reflect the tones in her stunning silver hair, as well as give them a more defined shape and color, we brushed a slate gray powder shadow through them. An ivory base shadow topped with a metallic taupe on the lids gave her eyes a natural lift. Black gel eyeliner layered with a smudged line of steel-gray shadow on the top lash line, combined with slate on the lower lash line, creates a soft, smoky effect that enhances Gro's sea-green eye color.

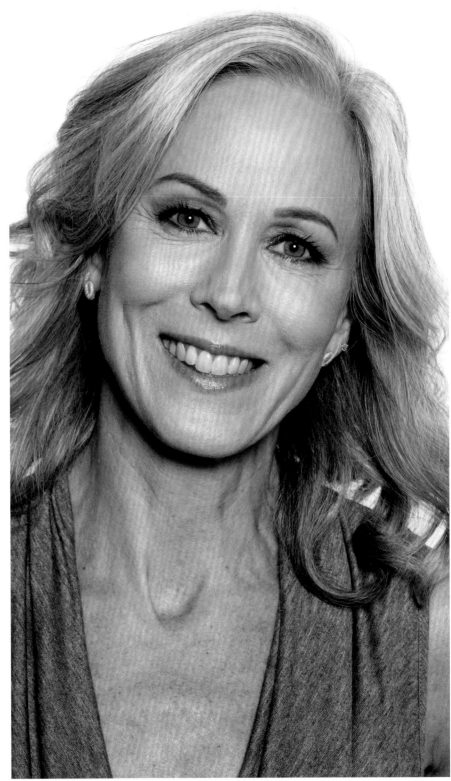

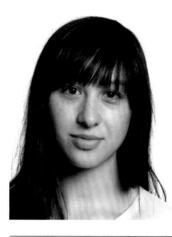

JANICE CHOU
FASHION CONTENT
COORDINATOR

*The best beauty advice I've fol-
lowed is actually a quote from
Full House: "The key to wearing
makeup is to not look like you're
wearing makeup."*

JANICE'S MAKEUP—
DAY

To even out Janice's skin, I spot-
applied a foundation stick where
she needed it with a foundation
brush, rubbing in the excess with
my fingers. I set her makeup with
a loose yellow-based powder
that neutralized any additional
redness. A combination of corrector and creamy concealer a
shade lighter than her skin tone
concealed undereye circles and
added brightness. A powder-
pink pot rouge provides a sheer
stained finish that looks beautiful
on Janice's lips and cheeks.

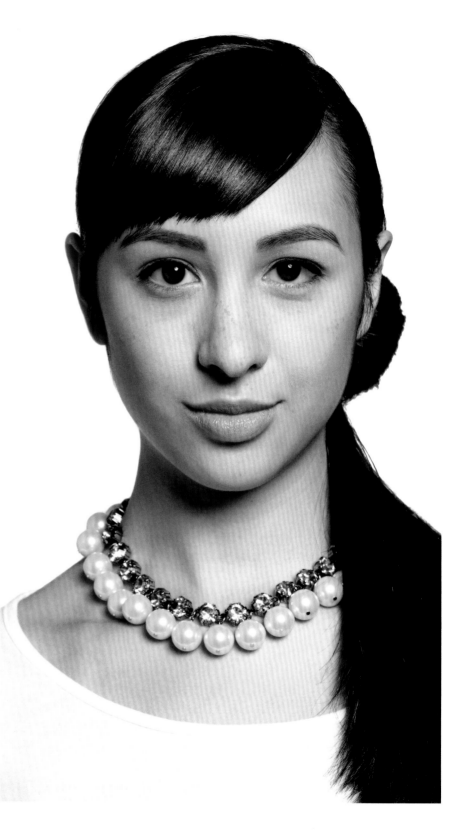

JANICE'S MAKEUP— NIGHT

Amping up Janice's eyes is what takes her look from day to night. I swept an ivory shadow all over her lids, followed by a matte purple shade from her lash line to just above the crease, layering shimmery purple eye shadow on top. For a party-ready look, I lined her top and bottom lashes with plum eye shadow. A heather-rose lipstick straight from the tube adds a neutral touch of pink to her gorgeous full lips.

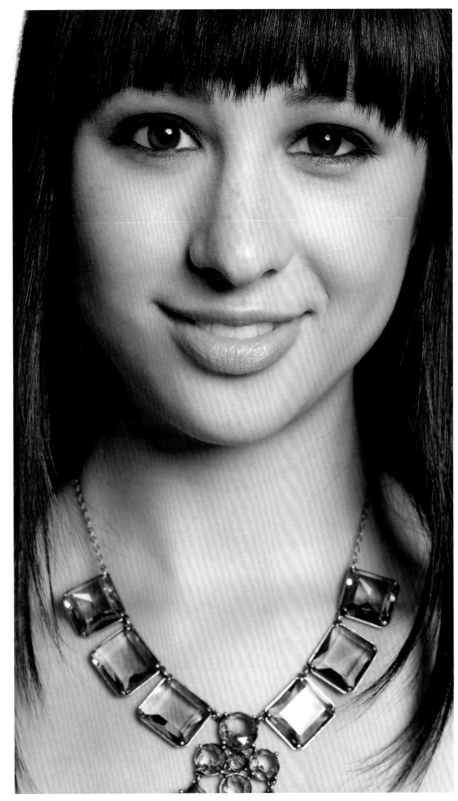

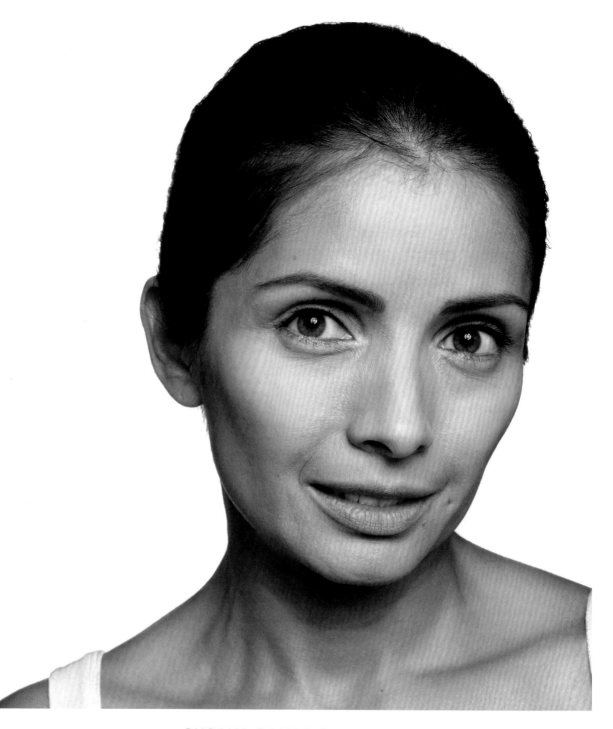

SUSANA CANARIO
FREELANCE MAKEUP ARTIST, MOTHER, WIFE
Stick foundation is my can't-live-without makeup item.

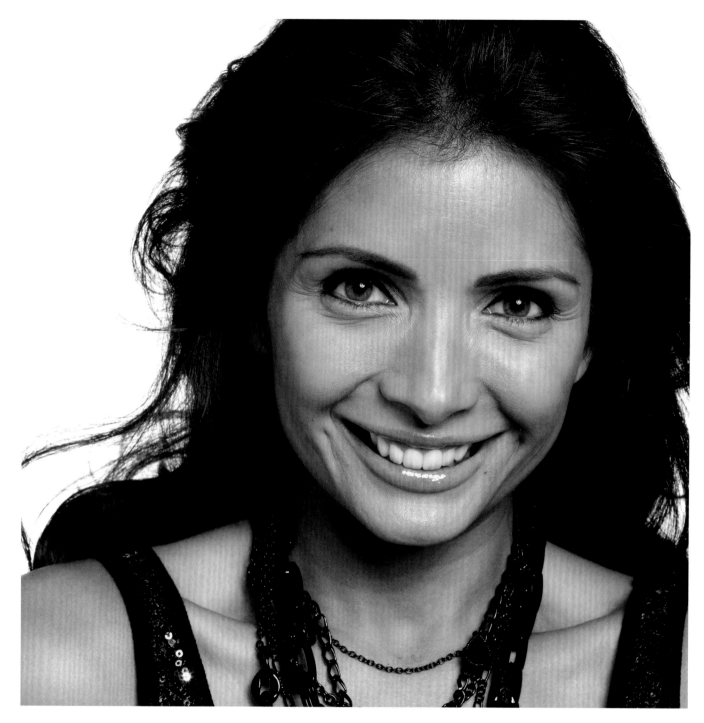

SUSANA'S MAKEUP

To warm up the skin, apply bronzer where the sun naturally hits your face—the forehead, cheeks, nose, chin, and neck. For a flushed, pretty color, I like to layer two shades of blush on top of bronzer—a blush that matches the color your cheeks turn when you exercise, in this case a tawny pink, with a pop of a brighter pale pink on the apples of the cheeks. A dab of face oil on cheeks gives Susana a gorgeous glow. To make Susana's eyes stand out, I drew a thick line of black gel liner along the top lashes, using the excess liner to trace a light line along the lower lash line for definition.

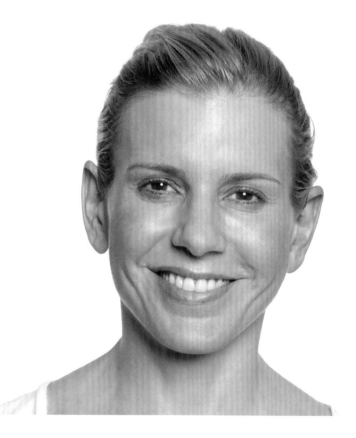

ALEXIS STEWART
AUTHOR, RADIO PERSONALITY

Alexis knows who she is. She is a strong woman who knows what she likes and what she wants, which I find really admirable. Alexis has grown up with an incredibly famous mother, Martha Stewart, but she is truly her own woman, and that really comes across when you meet her.

—

Alexis has been blessed with a beautiful face and dynamite body. To make Alexis's brown eyes pop, we applied a white shadow all over the lid, an espresso brown gel liner, and a few coats of black mascara.

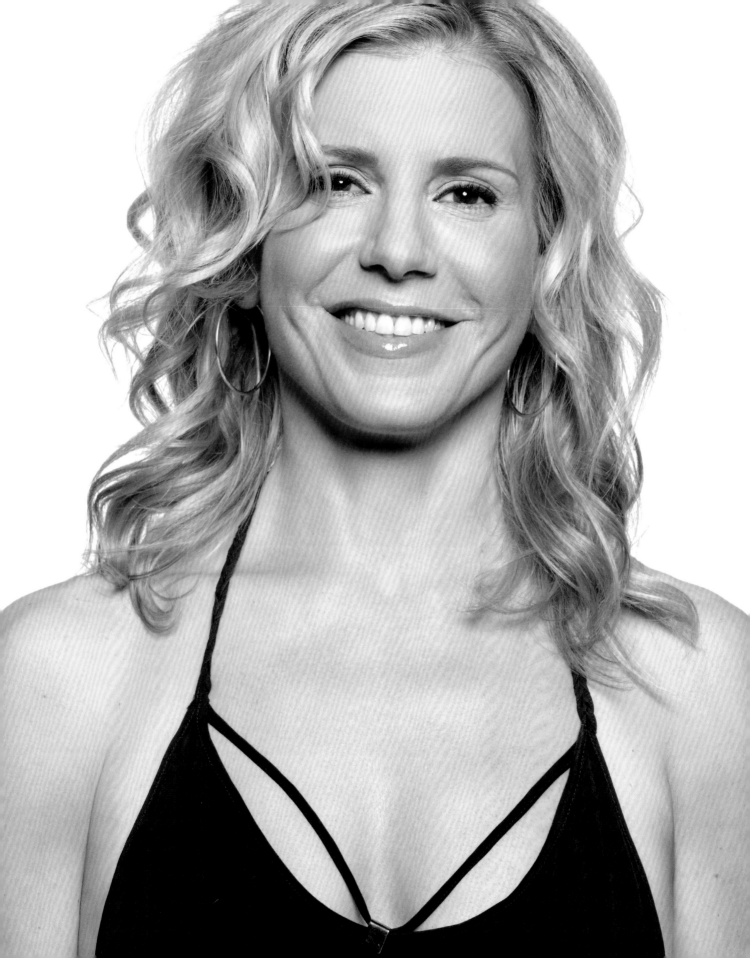

I've stayed out of the sun; that has been the best beauty advice I've ever gotten.

—ALEXIS STEWART

I recently had a daughter, so my greatest indulgence lately has been baby clothes, baby clothes, baby clothes! I turned into the person I said I would never be, and I buy very fancy baby clothes.

I want my daughter to be a lot of the things that I'm not. I want her to be comfortable. I was really shy and reserved, and I'm hoping that she won't be, because I think it is harder to be that way. Even if you just appear shy, it makes people think all kinds of things, like you're rude, and it's just because you're quiet and happy to sit back and watch rather than always join in and be the center of attention. I'm hoping she'll be a little more outgoing than I was; it will make her life easier.

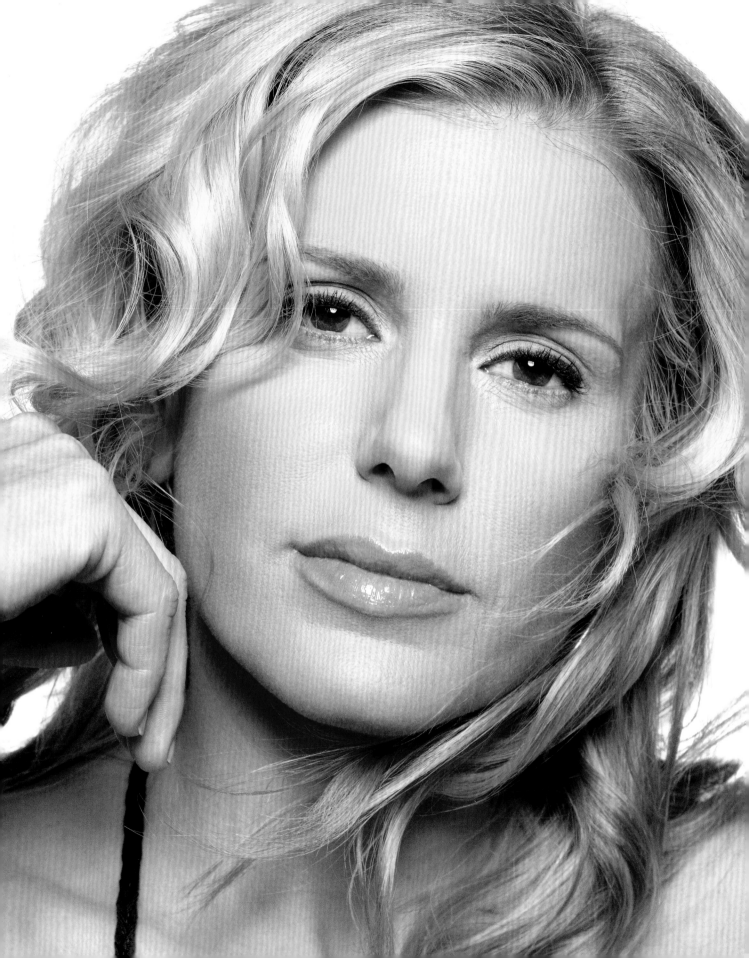

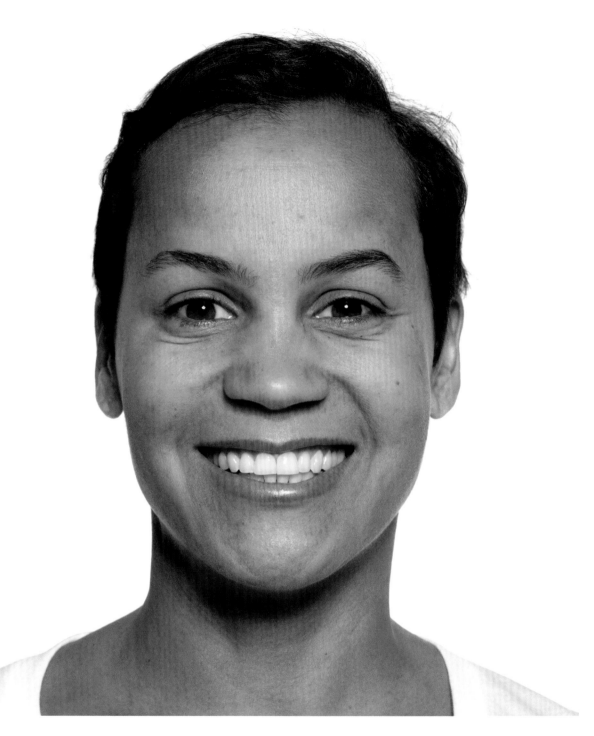

ERICA REID MOTHER

After my daughter and son were born, I went on a journey of self-rediscovery. I felt I had lost sight of who I was before I became a mom, so instead of wallowing, I took matters into my own hands. I gave myself a mini makeover; donated every last pair of sweatpants I owned; started working out; colored my hair; and then, as I got my mojo back, chopped off my locks to reveal this new, chic 'do!

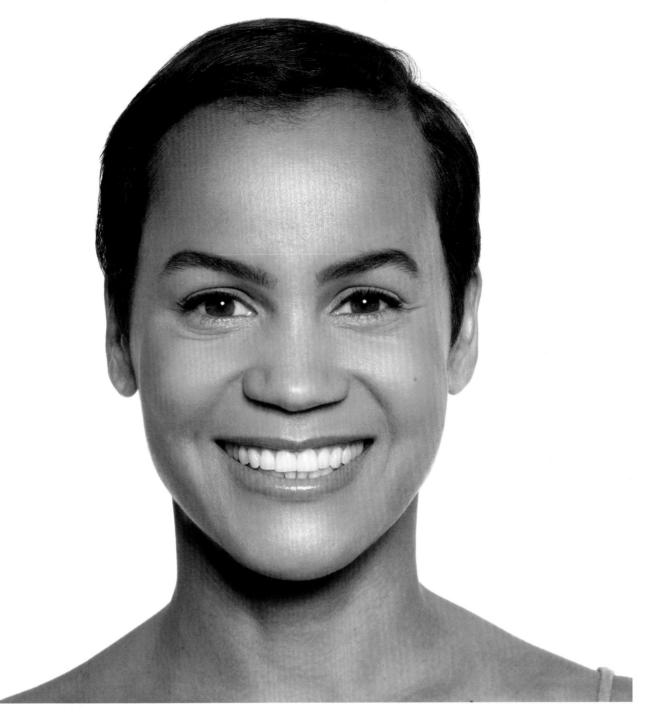

ERICA'S MAKEUP

To stay true to Erica's casual-chic style, we chose a gorgeous yet natural color palette for her eyes. We began by giving Erica's brows a polished look by using a brow brush and a mahogany shadow. For her lids, we applied an off-white shadow as a base and a taupe shadow in the crease for depth. To make eyes stand out, eyeliner should be always be darker than your eye color. For Erica, that meant going with a brownish-black gel liner that is a shade darker than her warm brown eyes.

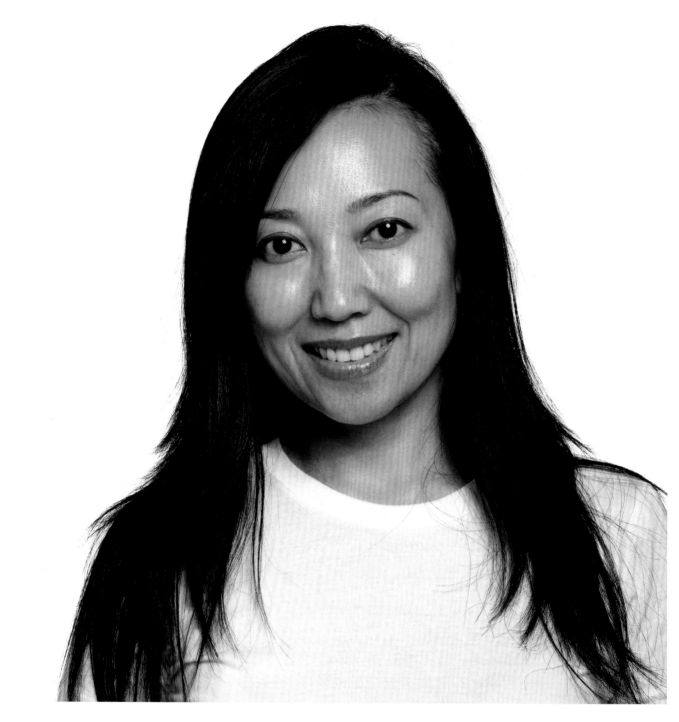

TINA CRAIG FASHION BLOGGER

*The best beauty advice I've gotten is from my grandma: Drink two glasses of
rainwater each morning on an empty stomach. Skin glows all day!*

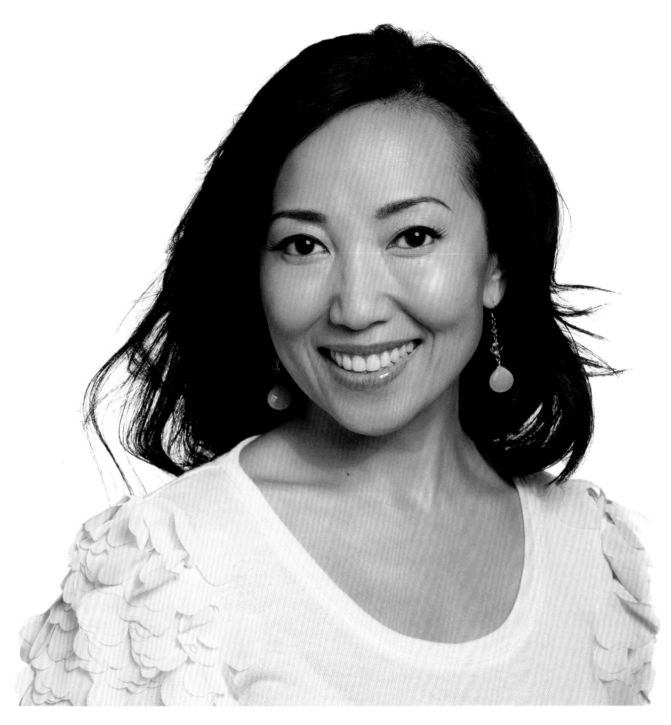

TINA'S MAKEUP

To complement Tina's radiant skin, I chose soft coral tones for eyes, lips, and cheeks. I love the subtle warmth of the coral pot rouge on her cheeks and lips and the hint of shimmer from the metallic peach eye shadow.

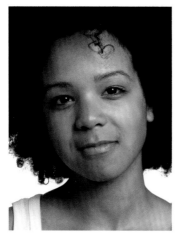

EVA PICHARDO
HAIRSTYLIST,
COLLEGE STUDENT

The thing that makes me feel beautiful on a bad day is having a flower in my hair.

EVA'S MAKEUP

We relied on soft, warm colors that complimented Eva's gorgeous skin to bring out her luminescence. When your lips have a lot of color like Eva's naturally pink pout, a lip gloss in the same shade is all you need for a radiant smile. An apricot blush on the apples of Eva's cheeks, blended up toward the hairline and then downward to soften any edges, gives her an illuminating pop of color. For eyes, we layered a banana shadow all over the lid and a warm bronze shimmer shadow applied from the lash line to just above the crease. Two coats of mascara, plus her signature flower in her hair, and Eva's ready to go.

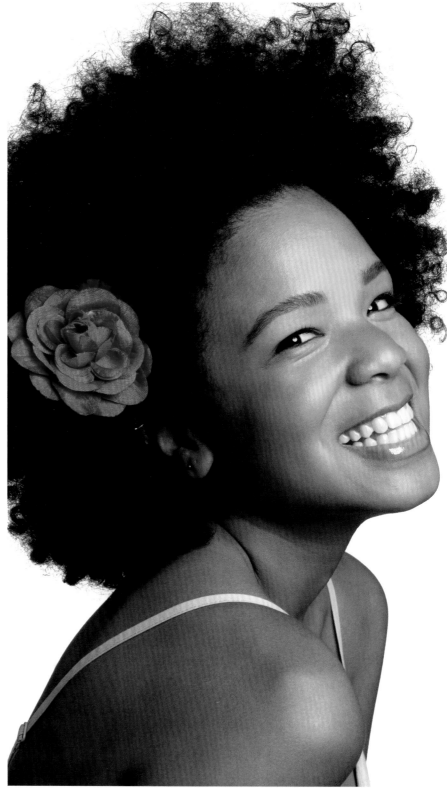

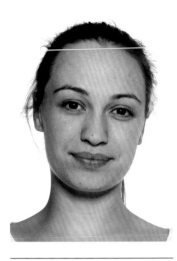

ALYSSA HULAHAN
MASSAGE
THERAPIST

It's amazing how the feature you perceive to be your worst can become your best. I used to get teased because of how big my lips were. Now, with everyone getting fillers and collagen, I feel lucky to have a perfect pout naturally.

ALYSSA'S MAKEUP

If you are blessed with large, expressive eyes like Alyssa's, it's important to keep liner thin and close to the lash line. This way eyes are defined but not over-powering. Curling Alyssa's lashes first followed by several coats of lengthening mascara highlights her eyes even more. To even out her complexion, we relied on a foundation stick applied with a sponge where needed and set with a yellow-based loose powder applied with a brush. Alyssa's full lips only need a touch of sheer gloss to make them shine.

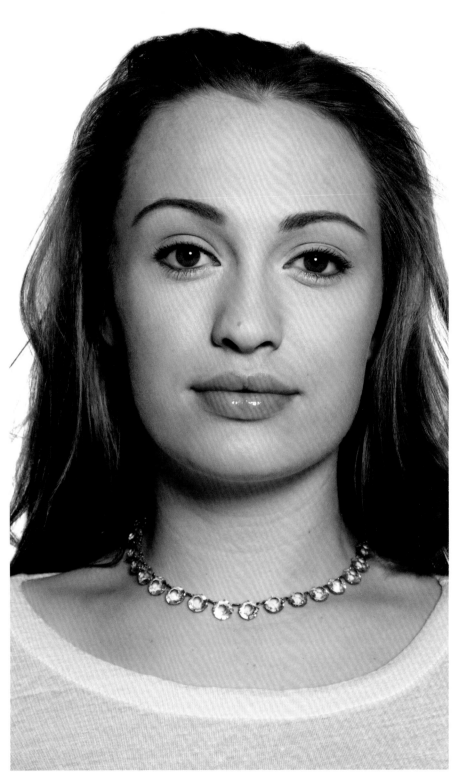

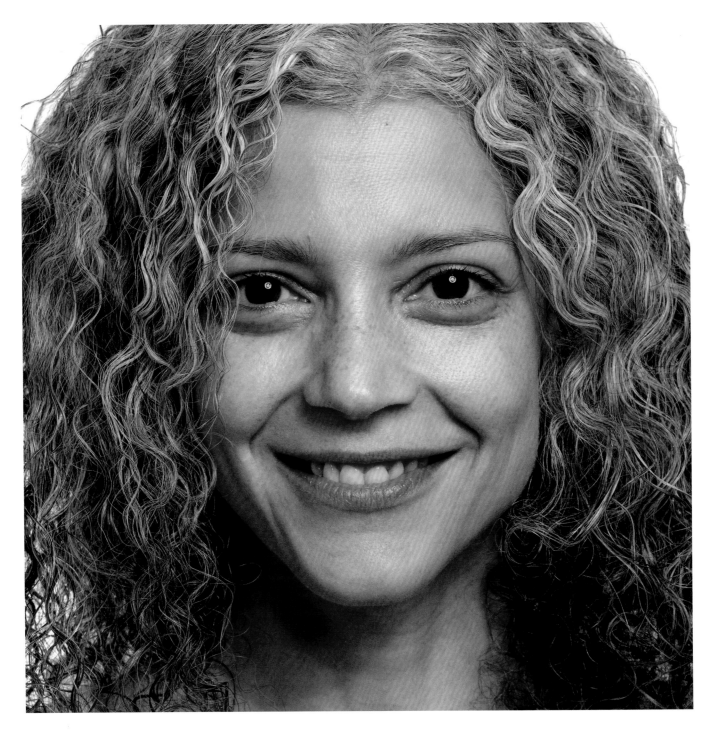

ROSANNE GUARARRA CREATIVE DIRECTOR

My mom taught me to moisturize every day and to never go to bed with makeup on.

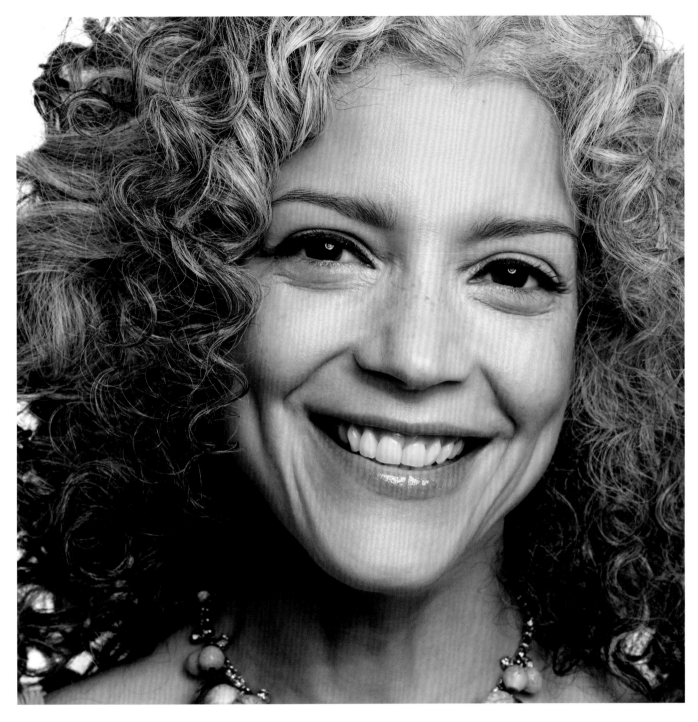

ROSANNE'S MAKEUP

When your hair goes gray, your face needs some extra color, and bright pinks and soft rose tones on cheeks and lips look amazing against Rosanne's gorgeous naturally curly hair. For Rosanne's eyes, we began by filling in brows using a dark brown shadow and a brow brush. White matte shadow applied to the lids followed by black gel liner and black mascara gives Rosanne a fresh, polished party look.

ALEXA RAY JOEL
ACTRESS, SINGER, SONGWRITER

———

I first met Alexa when she was a little girl. Alexa, the daughter of Christie Brinkley and Billy Joel, would have playdates with my son while I would do her mother's makeup. It's so cool to be doing Alexa's makeup now; I've watched her really come into her own. A few years ago I saw her perform with her dad and Bruce Springsteen in concert, and she floored everyone with her performance. Not only is she talented, and uniquely gorgeous, but also she is very open and warm.

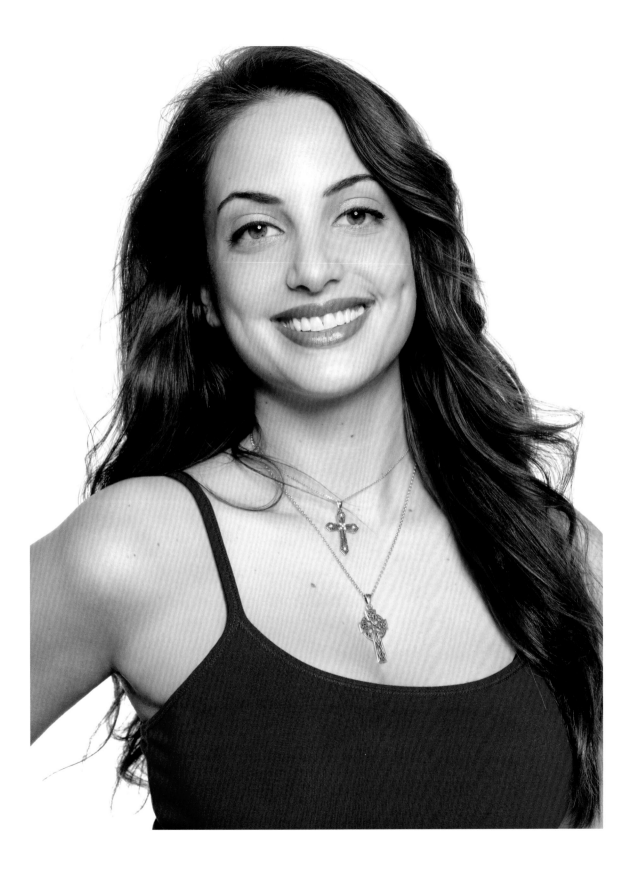

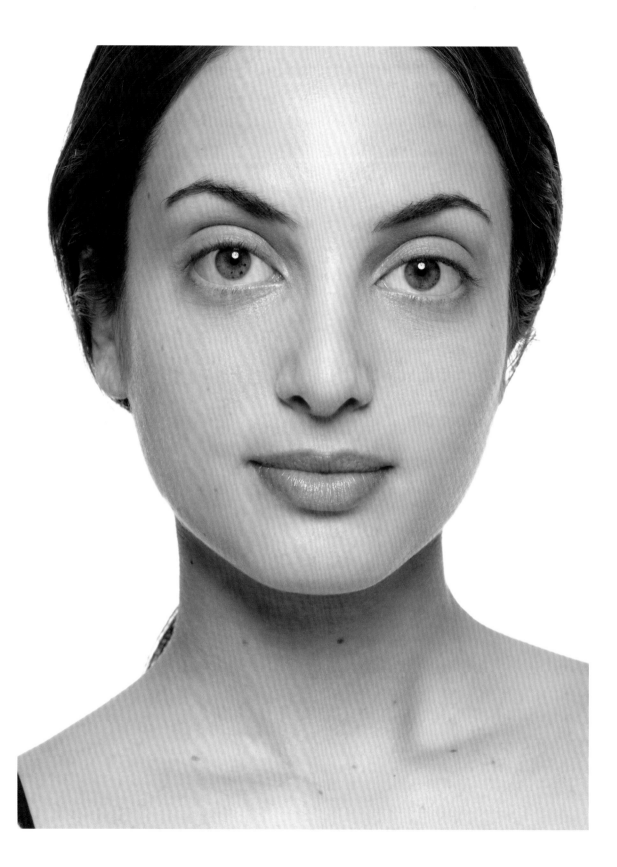

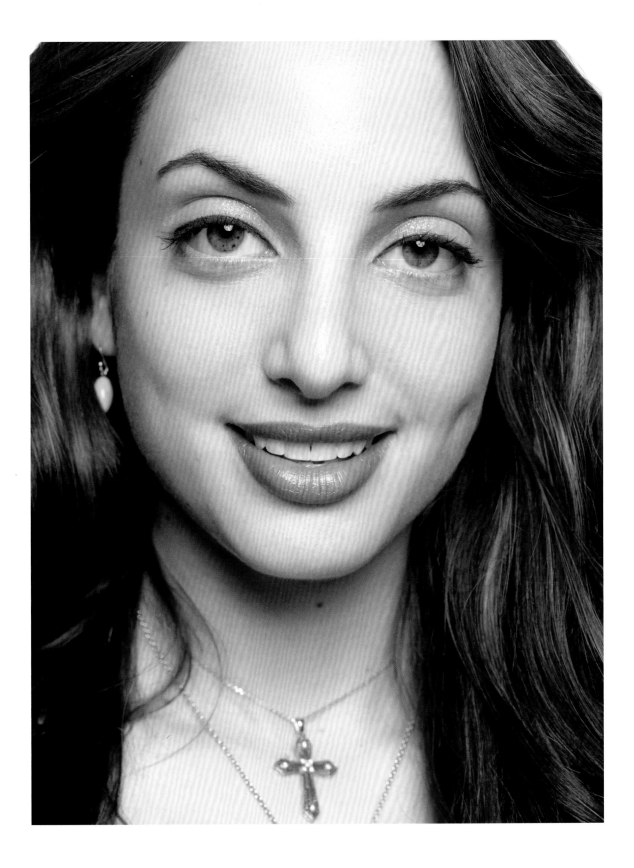

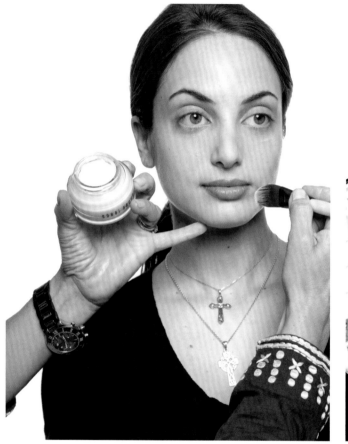

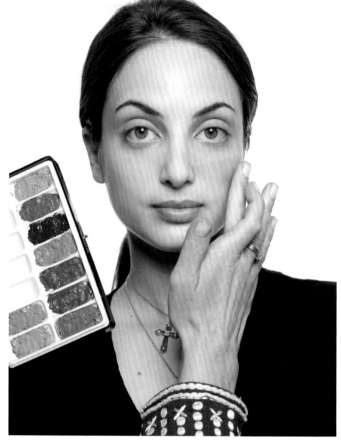

SKIN

Applying a hydrating face cream instantly makes skin appear more vibrant. Alexa only needed a touch of foundation, to even out redness. After a little corrector and concealer under the eyes, she was ready for color.

CHEEKS

To give Alexa's cheeks some pop, I blended a creamy blush in the perfect washed pink tone from the apples of her cheeks to her hairline.

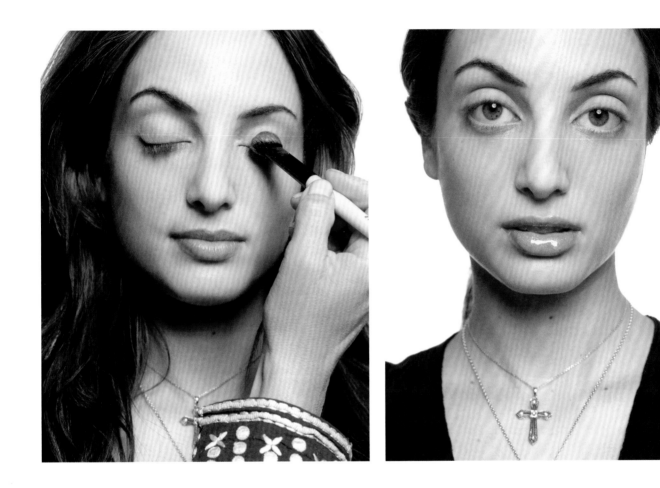

EYES

Because Alexa has really expressive eyes, she only needs a light color shadow to spotlight their great shape. A dense eye shadow brush deposits enough light ivory powder for a polished look.

DAYTIME LIPS

Alexa has incredible, full lips, so she doesn't need lip liner. Instead, a peachy-pink shimmer gloss gives her a sweet, natural look.

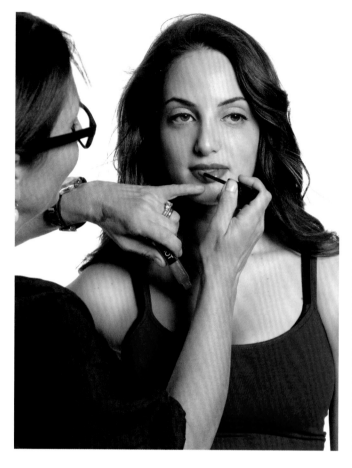

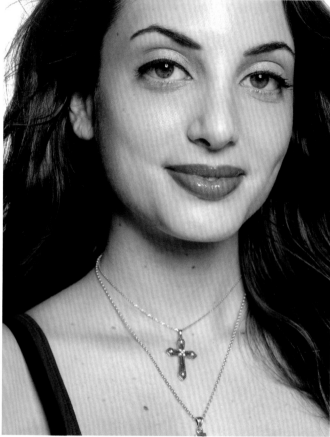

NIGHTTIME LIPS

Alexa loves color, so I thought it would be beautiful to do a red-pink gloss on her lips for nighttime. The gloss is transparent and looks really fresh and modern.

EVENING EYES

Sheer shimmery shadows in very subtle shades of champagne and platinum, paired with a sweep of black gel liner and several coats of mascara, give Alexa's eyes a captivating yet understated look.

We all do things to try to look pretty. But if that isn't complemented with inner beauty, it is such a waste.

—ALEXA RAY JOEL

I like the feeling when I've written a song that I can feel really inside of and really believe in. It's this huge high, this real energy rush. I think that is the goal for all art: that it be fluid and natural and come from a very real deep part of your soul.

My teenage years were rough. I was painfully shy. I was terrified of boys. I was a really late bloomer. I had my first kiss when I was seventeen or eighteen. When I was nineteen, I went to NYU and started performing in their musical theater program. You have to build confidence and accept yourself if you are going to get up on that stage and give it your all. It's so much easier when you love yourself. I'm not shy any more.

I went through some traumatic stuff in the media. When you've been heartbroken and you've had everybody see you when you're in a difficult state like that, it does toughen you up. It makes you go, *Hey, I'm not perfect!* As a result you feel more beautiful because you're like, *You know what? You just saw me at my most vulnerable point.* It is just life. It happens and I've learned to get through it.

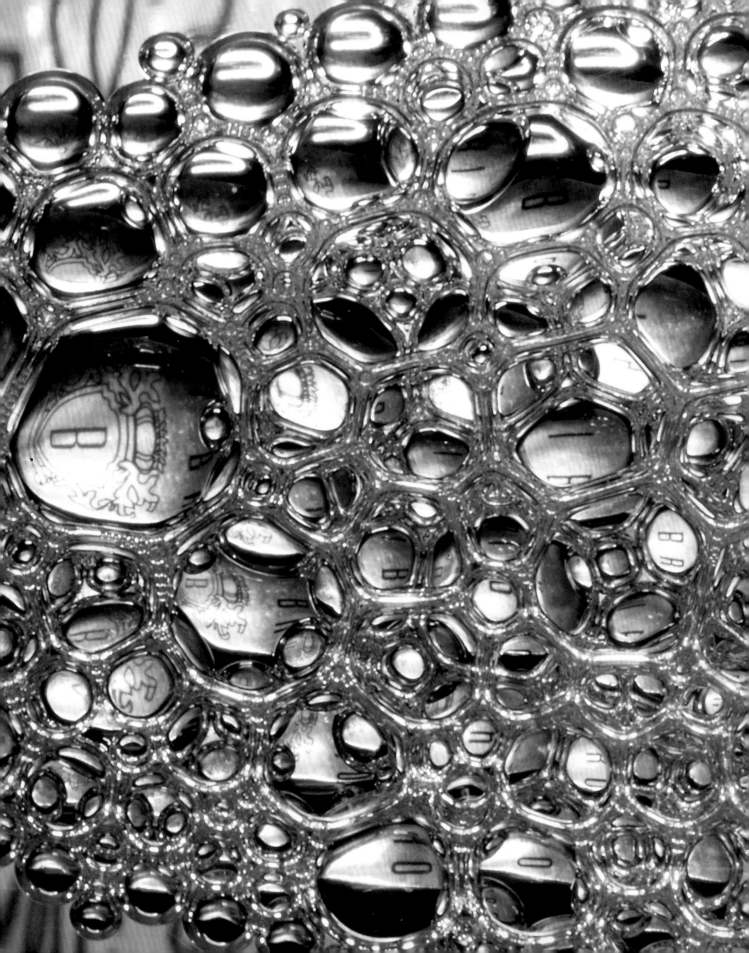

03

PRETTY STRONG

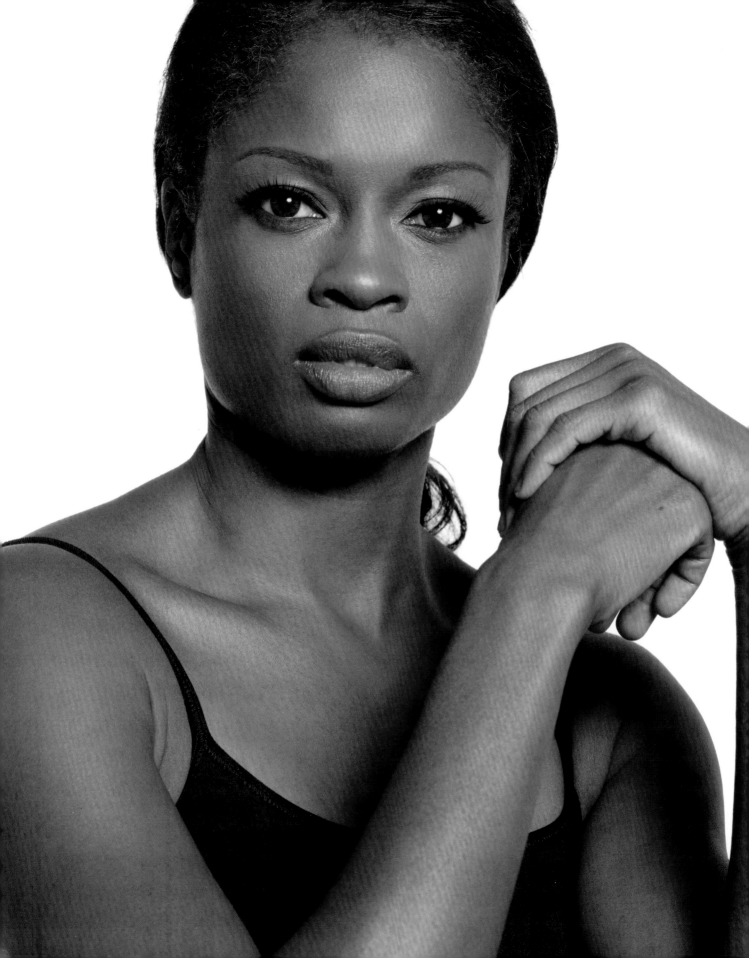

PRETTY STRONG

A woman can be strong in character or strong in body. When both qualities come together, as they do in many of the women in this chapter, it is pretty powerful. The women featured here make a living through exercise, either by empowering others as trainers and motivators, or as competitors themselves. They are at the top of their game and incredibly inspiring. I've been lucky enough to work with dozens of athletes over the years from Billie Jean King to Venus Williams. I am in awe of their positive attitude and determination to keep forging ahead no matter what the circumstances. They are examples to us all.

Most people don't realize that female professional athletes are judged not only on their competitive skills, but also on how they look. They have to be on camera frequently, sometimes after a grueling workout. Their livelihoods often depend on promoting products. These athletes truly understand how to make themselves the best they can possibly be—through fitness, beauty, mental endurance, a healthy lifestyle, and a winning attitude. One of the most important things I've learned from athletes is to think of food as fuel. Athletes choose to eat what will make them strong, and it is such a positive, healthy way to view food. They exemplify the idea of mind over body on a daily basis. I know there are days when these women don't feel pretty and don't feel their best. Even athletes have moments when they would rather sit one out than get on the field. On those days, however, they do what we should all do—put our hair in a ponytail, lace up our sneakers, and get out there. I admire Pretty Strong women because they exemplify the awesome Nike slogan *Just Do It*.

BEING STRONG

Beauty tips for women on the run

———

DAY

SKIN

Sunscreen is essential. If you're an athlete who trains and competes outside, you will need a heavy-duty, waterproof, long-lasting product that has an SPF between 25 and 50. Your sunscreen should be on par with what a lifeguard wears, not your average moisturizing version.

To even out skin tone, tinted moisturizer is the best choice for athletes. It soaks into skin, won't look heavy or out of place, and stays on.

Long-wear concealer keeps dark circles at bay for hours. Avoid products that are so moisturizing they melt off at first sweat, or so drying so that you can see every eye crease. You need a product with just the right balance.

CHEEKS

Runners and high-endurance athletes seldom need blush, as their cheeks naturally flush. For golfers and yogis, a sweep of powder blush enhances a nice healthy glow.

EYES

For eyes, choose long-lasting products that can stand up to sweat—gel liner and waterproof mascara.

LIPS

Just touch of gloss or lip balm is all you need for lips.

HAIR

Whether you are swimming or competing outdoors, you need to take extra care of your hair to keep it healthy and strong. Deep conditioning helps moisturize, protect, and strengthen your hair. Short styles, cuts that keep hair away from the face, or a reliable ponytail will let you keep moving while looking great.

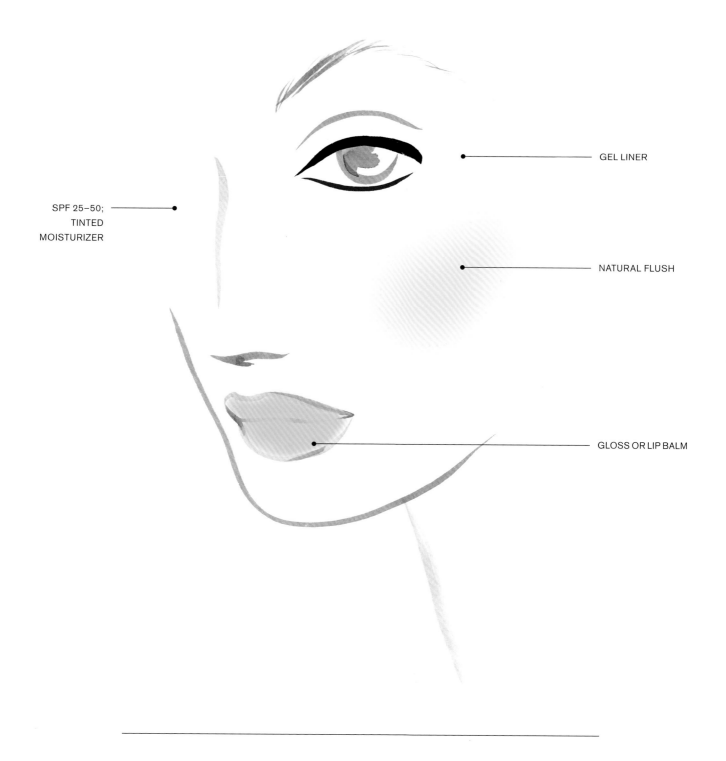

GEL LINER

SPF 25–50;
TINTED
MOISTURIZER

NATURAL FLUSH

GLOSS OR LIP BALM

BEING STRONG

Keep it natural, but have some fun

———

EVENING

SKIN

At night you can be free of the long-wear formulas and heavy SPF creams and let your skin breathe a bit. Light foundation or a tinted moisturizer, paired with corrector and concealer underneath eyes, provides a pretty base and a natural freshness that suits active women beautifully.

CHEEKS

For evening you want healthy rosy cheeks that echo the flush you get when you are active. A sweep of natural blush paired with shimmer on the apples of cheeks enhances your luminescence.

EYES

Athletes don't get to play with eye makeup during the day, so for night you should have fun with your makeup. A sexy, yet soft, smoky eye easily takes you from sporty to glamorous.

LIPS

Especially with a smokier eye, keep lips and cheeks ultra-feminine with rosy pink shades for both. There is a natural beauty that comes from taking care of your body, and pretty, soft makeup plays that up without overpowering your healthy look.

HAIR

At night, it is all about saying good-bye to the practical ponytail and any holders that keep your hair in place while you work out. Instead, let your hair down. Give it some soft waves or a glam blowout. You'll still look like you, though, just with a feminine, pretty style.

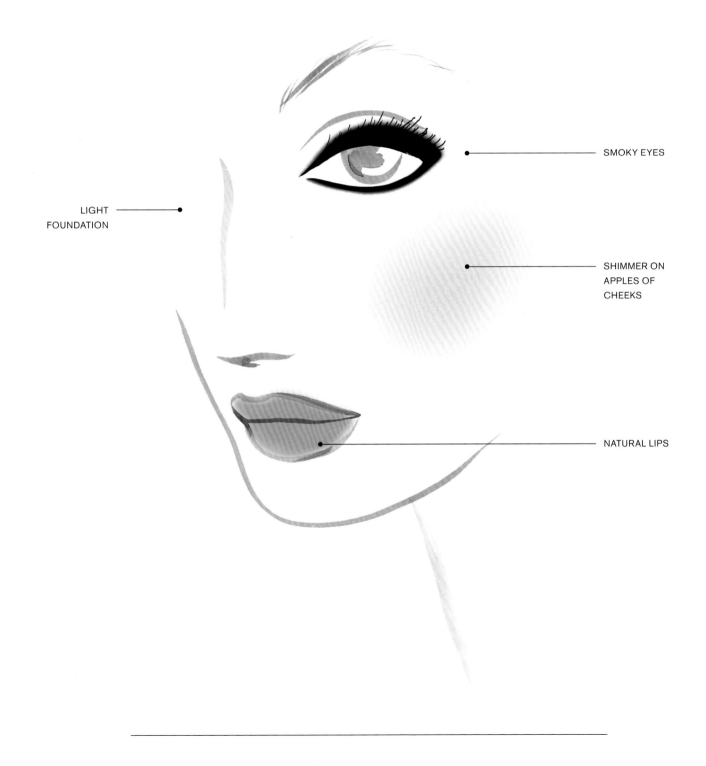

SMOKY EYES

LIGHT
FOUNDATION

SHIMMER ON
APPLES OF
CHEEKS

NATURAL LIPS

KEISHER McLEOD-WELLS

A.K.A. FIRE, THE BOXING DIVA.
PROFESSIONAL BOXER

———

Keisher caught my attention when she was profiled in the *New York Times.* I love when people do things you don't expect, and you don't usually read about a slight girl who looks like a model but is actually a professional boxer. Keisher has more than a dozen championships under her belt and wants to win a World Championship title. One of the things I noticed immediately about Keisher was how sweet and feminine she is. I like that she feels as comfortable being a girly girl as she does showing off her strength in the ring.

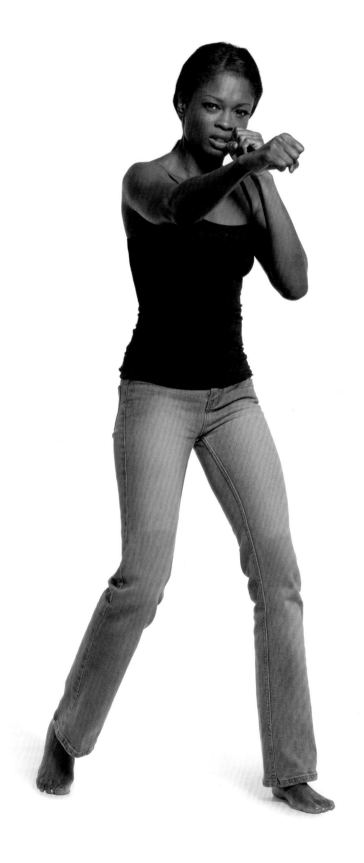

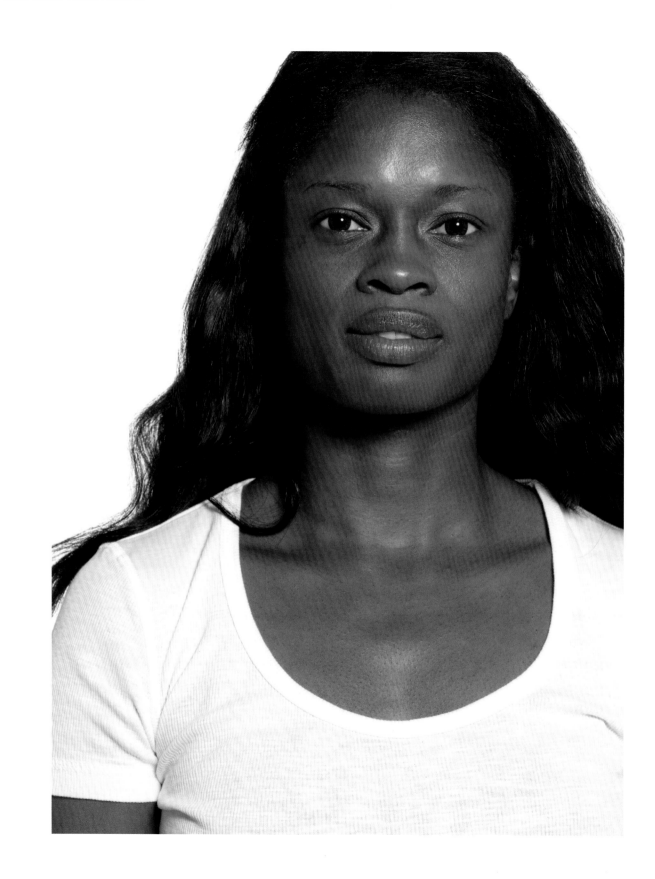

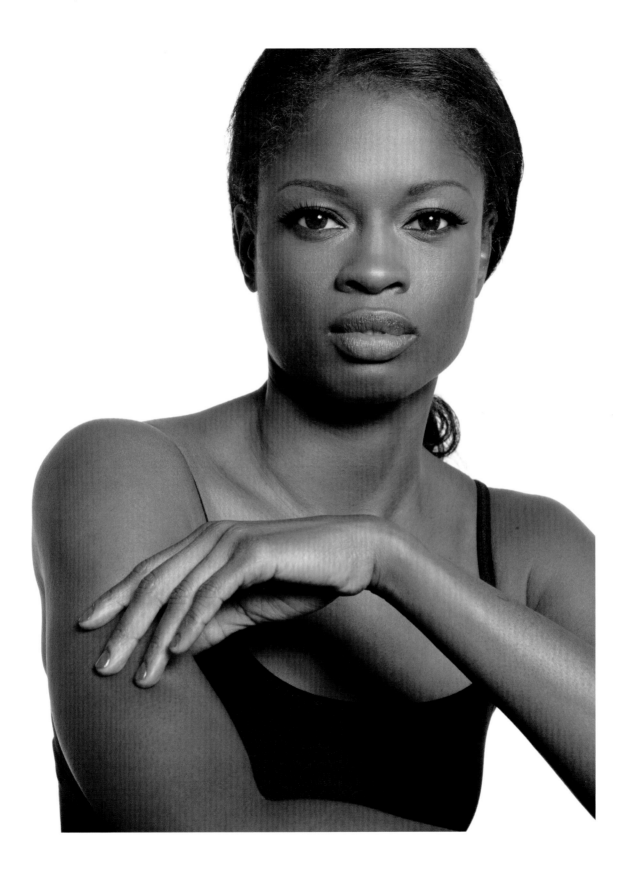

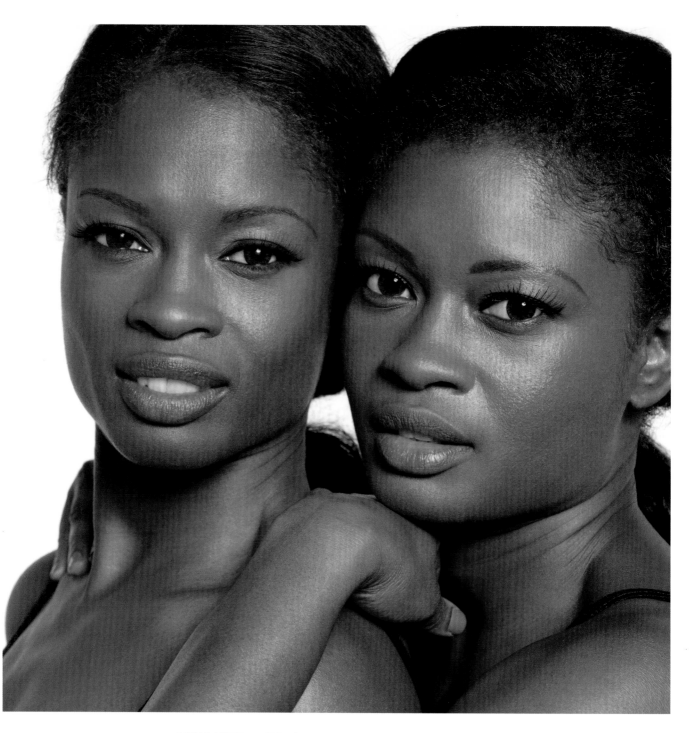

KEISHER & TEISHER McLEOD'S MAKEUP

The twin sisters have such striking features they really don't need a lot of makeup to stand out. I focused on defining their eyes with espresso and black liner, curling their amazing long lashes, and applying a couple of coats of mascara. To complete their look, I relied on just a touch of bronzer and clear lip balm.

The best piece of advice I've gotten is to not judge a book by its cover.

—KEISHER McLEOD-WELLS

Not in my wildest dreams did I think I would become a boxer. I was acting and modeling for years. But when a trainer told me I should think about competing, I just said yes without even thinking about it. My first fight was very scary. I was very nervous. But when I went in the ring, the nerves just disappeared and I won! I don't think I got touched one time.

Being accepted in this sport as someone so feminine, I've had to prove a lot. In the gym I wasn't taken seriously in the beginning. It took a little bit to overcome, but I worked hard and became very well respected in the boxing community.

The best piece of advice I've gotten is to not judge a book by its cover. People tend to think of boxers as one stereotype. But I've learned not to judge. I apply it to my life outside of boxing as well.

After a victory I'm at my highest adrenaline level. Especially after a tough fight, I'm feeling like I'm on top of the world and I have all the power.

FOOD IS FUEL

I recently read an article in which an actress described what she ate to stay thin. It was coffee for breakfast, salad with protein for lunch, and a dinner of steamed veggies and fish. It sounds more like starvation than a diet. I'm not a naturally thin person and I've tried many approaches to maintain my weight. Most of them just didn't leave me feeling good. A yogurt for lunch? I'm hungry a few hours (or minutes) later. Trend diets? Impossible to maintain.

What works for me is eating food that fills me up, is rich in nutrients, and most important, fuels my body. This means eating as many vegetables as possible, a bit of fruit, a small amount of protein, and a few complex carbs. I've also discovered raw fiber keeps me full. I put nine grams of fiber in a protein shake in the morning and I'm energized and not hungry (it's also a great trick before going to a party). If I focus on the bigger picture and eating really well most of the time, I can enjoy occasionally going off the plan. I've learned the building blocks for a strong, powerful body truly come from what you eat.

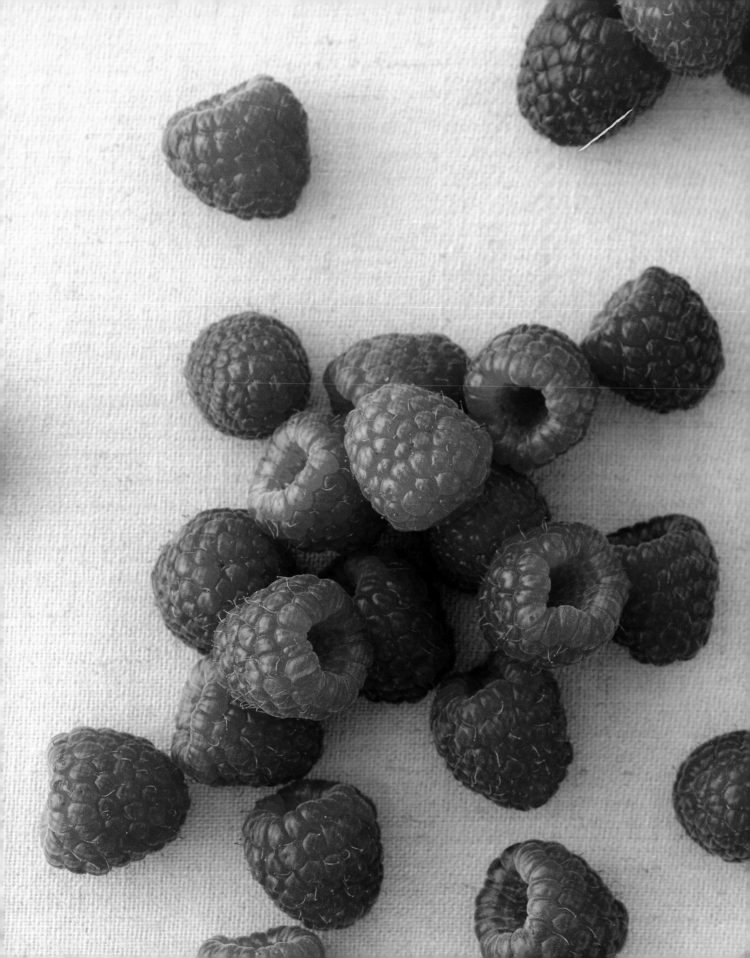

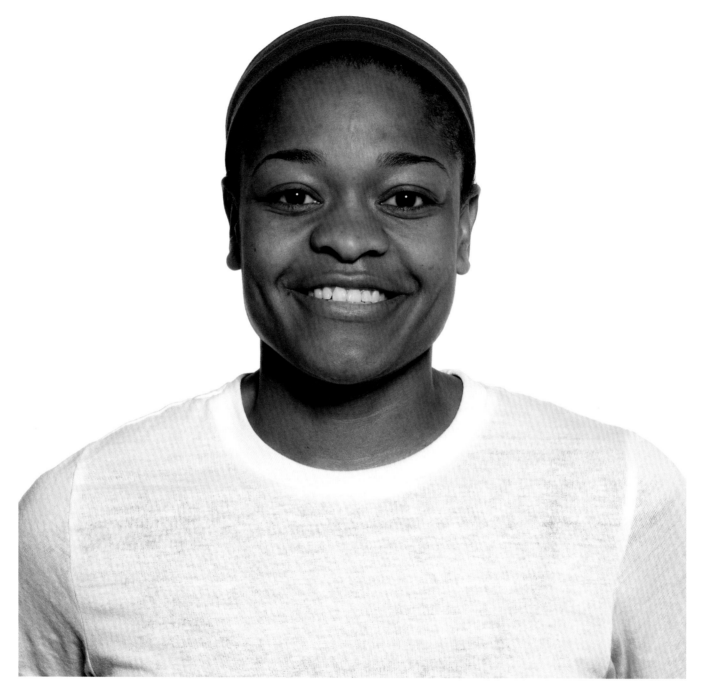

ALANA MONIQUE BEARD
PROFESSIONAL BASKETBALL PLAYER

*I like that I can be versatile. I can dress up completely or dress down in sweats,
a T-shirt, and no makeup and feel confident in my appearance.*

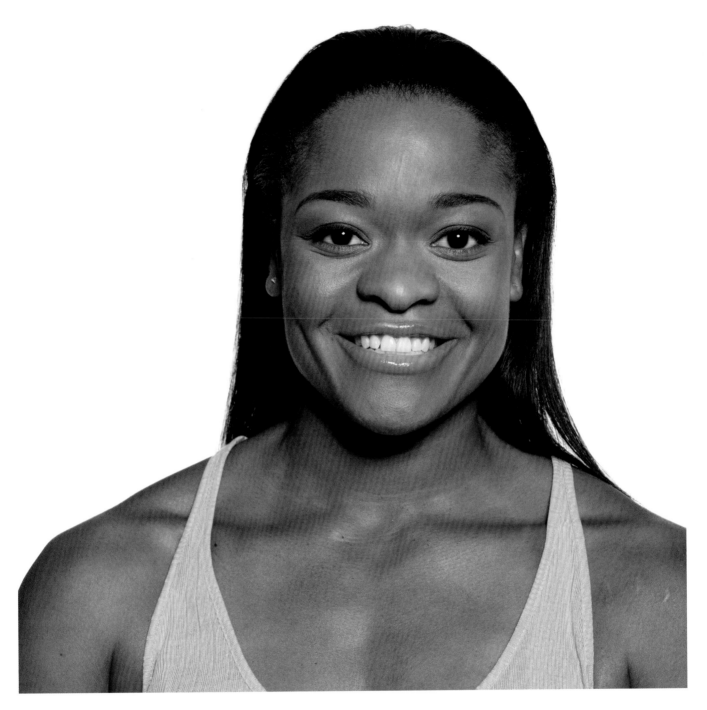

ALANA'S MAKEUP

To warm up Alana's beautiful skin, we applied a liquid foundation in an almond shade topped with a light dusting of soft brown sheer pressed powder. Bronzer on her cheeks, forehead, nose, chin, and neck, paired with a pop of apricot blush, brought out the pretty peach undertones in her skin. To complement her cheeks, we chose a pale peach lip color and a clear gloss for lips. We highlighted Alana's almond-shaped eyes with a medium purple metallic cream shadow applied all over the lid, with a layer of deep plum shimmer shadow on top.

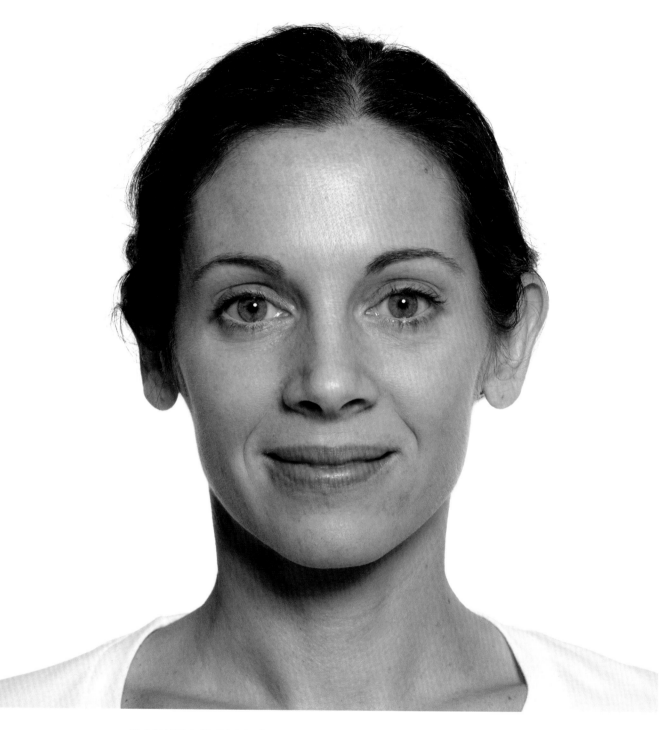

DANIELLE DIAMOND YOGA INSTRUCTOR, WRITER

It's the little things—yoga retreats, being told I look beautiful by my husband (even on those no-makeup days), ice cream, and mastering a perfect handstand—that make life worth living.

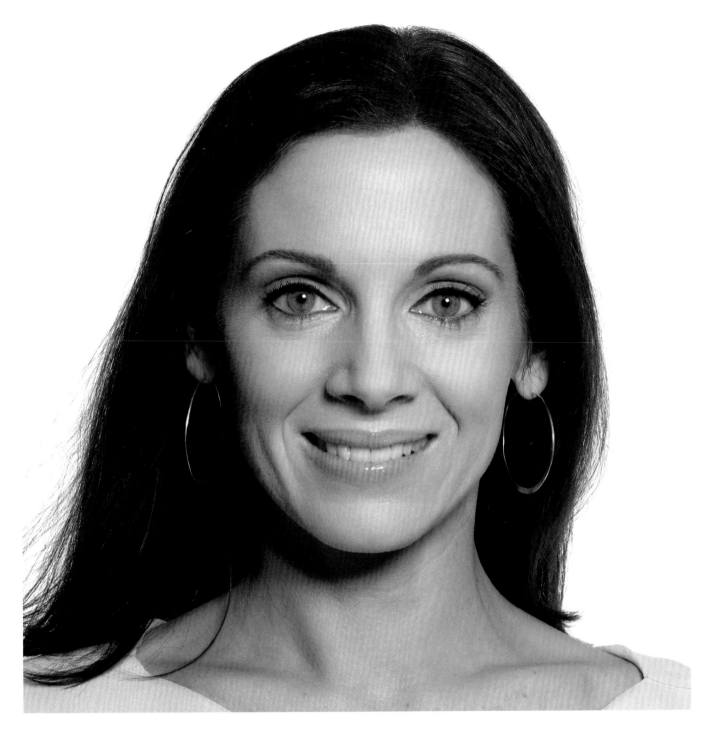

DANIELLE'S MAKEUP

I put the spotlight on Danielle's captivating blue eyes with bone and heather-purple shades over the lid. The soft purple shade sets off rather than competes with blue eyes. Black liquid gel liner on the top lash line with a softer line on the bottom adds definition. I kept lips and cheeks soft with natural shades of pink.

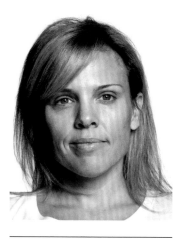

JENNIFER KOHL
YOGA INSTRUCTOR

My favorite feature is my smile because it's genuine.

JENNIFER'S MAKEUP

To bring out Jennifer's cool personality and stunning blue eyes, I swept an ivory shadow over the entire lid, layering a metallic ice-silver shadow from the lash line to just above the crease. To catch the light, I put the same sparkly shade in the inner corner of her eyes. This is a good trick if you want to bring some extra dazzle to your look, day or night.

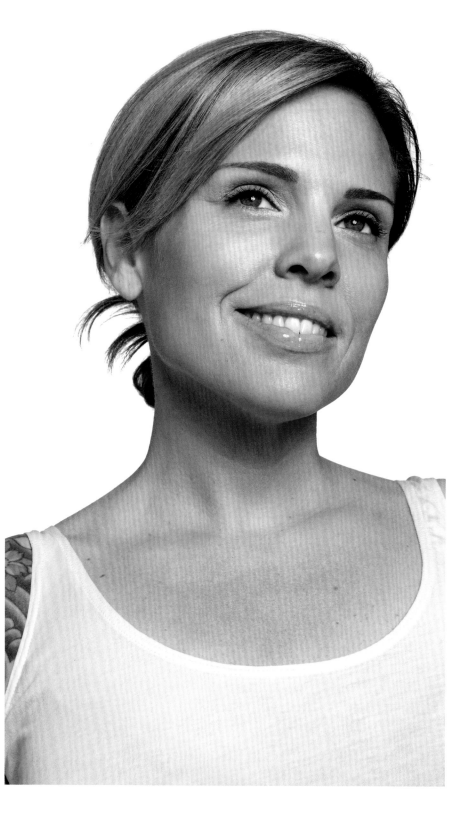

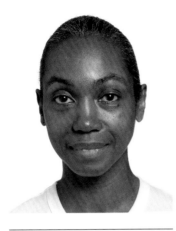

CRYSTAL GAYNOR
FITNESS TRAINER

The best compliment that I've ever received is that I radiate beauty from the outside and inside.

CRYSTAL'S MAKEUP

Crystal is over fifty, amazingly fit, and gorgeous. To capture how hip and youthful she is, we went with a statement lip in a rich mahogany shade that looks incredible with her skin tone. If you have beautiful chocolate-plum lips like Crystal, you can go with a dramatic dark color for a look that is cool and not goth.

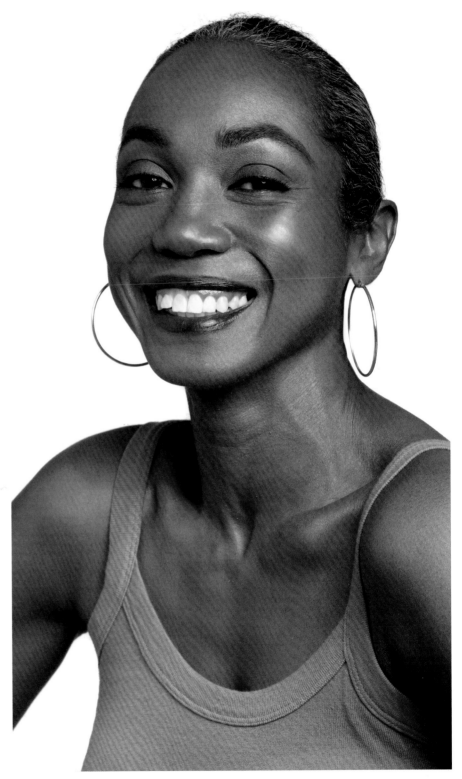

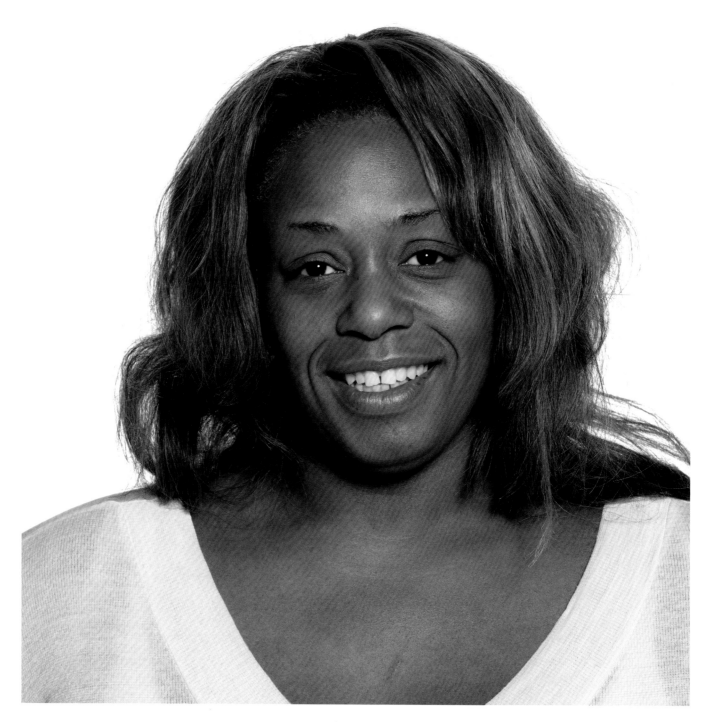

ANGEL WILLIAMS ENTERTAINER, FITNESS INSTRUCTOR

As I'm transforming my body through dance and exercise, tightening and toning my physical self, I'm also working to resurrect my soul from the baggage I've carried around in the past. No matter how I look, confidence is my most beautiful attribute. I'm attractive because I like myself and it shows.

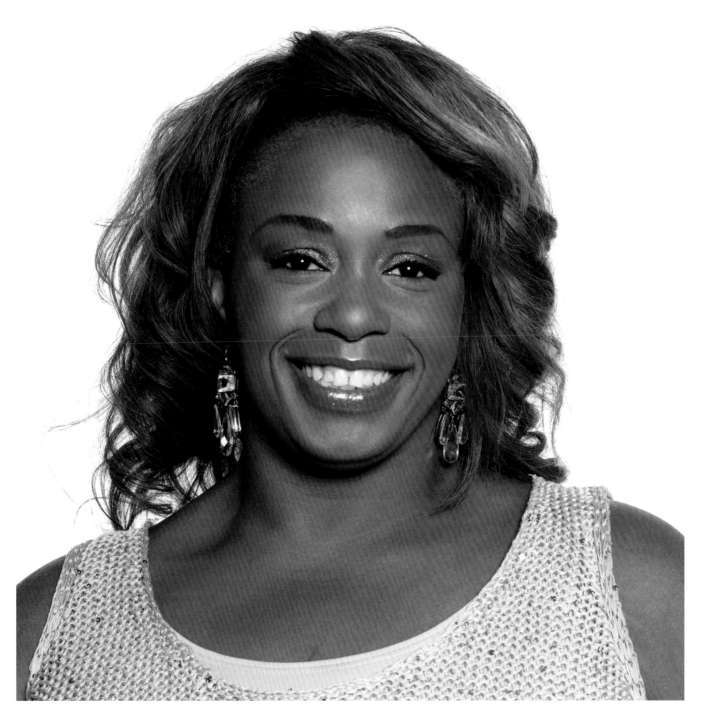

ANGEL'S MAKEUP

Angel has incredible energy and a natural sparkle that we enhanced with touches of shimmer on her eyes and lips. To create the look of perfect arched brows, we used a brow brush to sweep a rich brown shadow across the entire arch in short, feathery strokes. A toasted-peach shadow applied underneath her brow bone further defines her brows. To give her eyes the star treatment, we relied on a glittery cream shadow on her lids and a thick line of black gel eyeliner smudged with a plum shimmer shadow liner on top. Cranberry blush provides a natural flush that works beautifully with Angel's skin tone.

KEEPING IT MOVING

The day I graduated college, I made two big changes in my life—I quit smoking and I decided to start exercising. I was in my early twenties and I came to the realization that I didn't want to be an unhealthy person. It was around the time that *Self* magazine launched, and it talked a lot about how looking good and feeling good went hand in hand. The message really influenced me. *Self* also put athletic brunettes on the cover, and it made me think, *I might not look like Cheryl Tiegs, but I can be a healthy, athletic, Bobbi kind of woman.*

Having never exercised before, I started out by trying everything that was popular at the time—weight lifting, high-impact aerobics, and of course the Jane Fonda workout. Today, I do a mix of running, weights, yoga, boot camp, and spinning. I opened my own spinning studio near my house, because I think it is such an incredible workout. The variety keeps exercise fun and not boring. It's such a part of my life I can't imagine not working out. Being active keeps me strong, relieves stress, and makes me feel unstoppable (and it's the best beauty secret I have). My advice if you want to start is to just get out there and try everything you can. Whether it's walking or skiing or swimming, the key is finding that activity that inspires you to get off the couch and get moving.

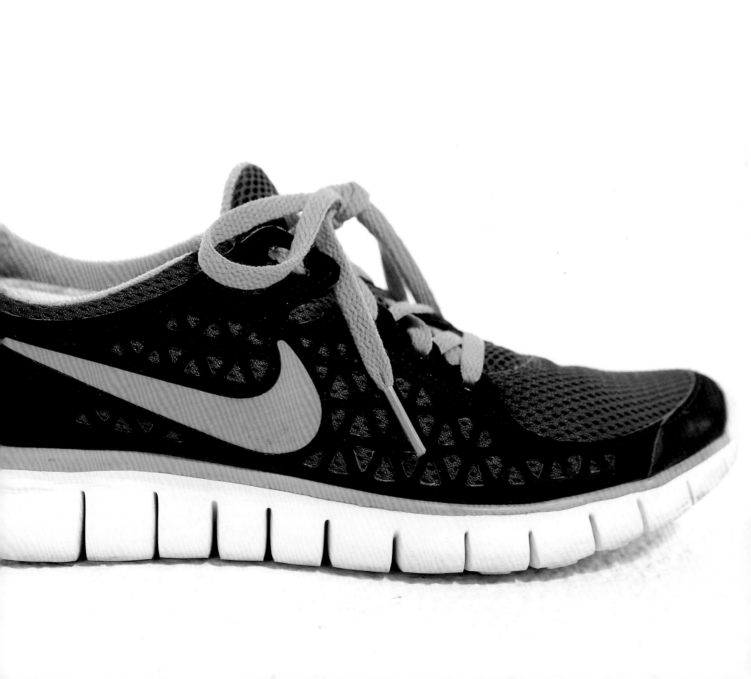

CRISTIE KERR
&
NATALIE GULBIS
PROFESSIONAL GOLFERS

———

Cristie and Natalie are professional golfers who have both undergone their own evolutions while in the spotlight. Natalie spent years wearing very strong makeup, but I've encouraged her to let her real beauty shine through. She now sports a more low-key look that still shows off her glamorous side. Cristie devoted herself to a healthful lifestyle a few years back and lost more than seventy pounds. Cristie's game has never been better, and her new confidence shows. Cristie and Natalie take pride in being role models for female athletes. They have devoted themselves to not only being great at their sport, but also to using their platform to support charities and inspire young girls.

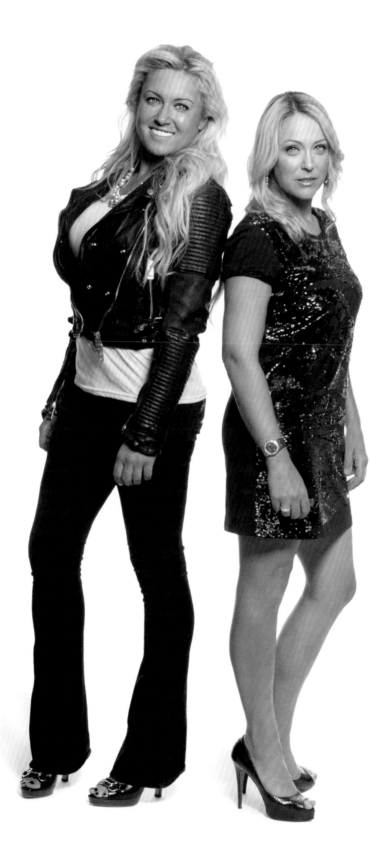

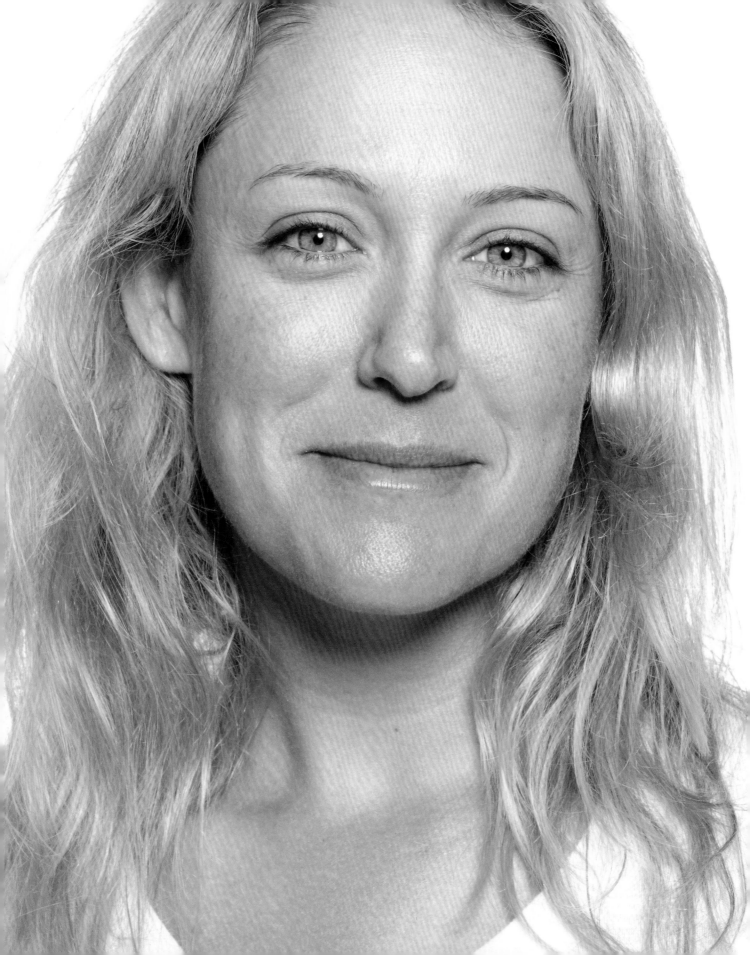

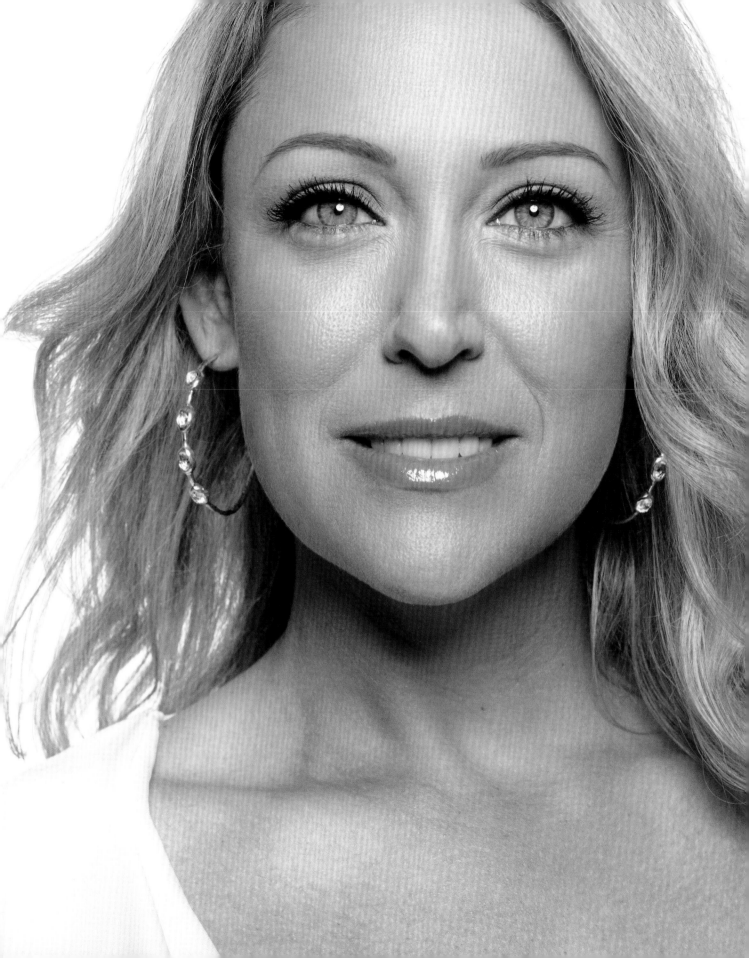

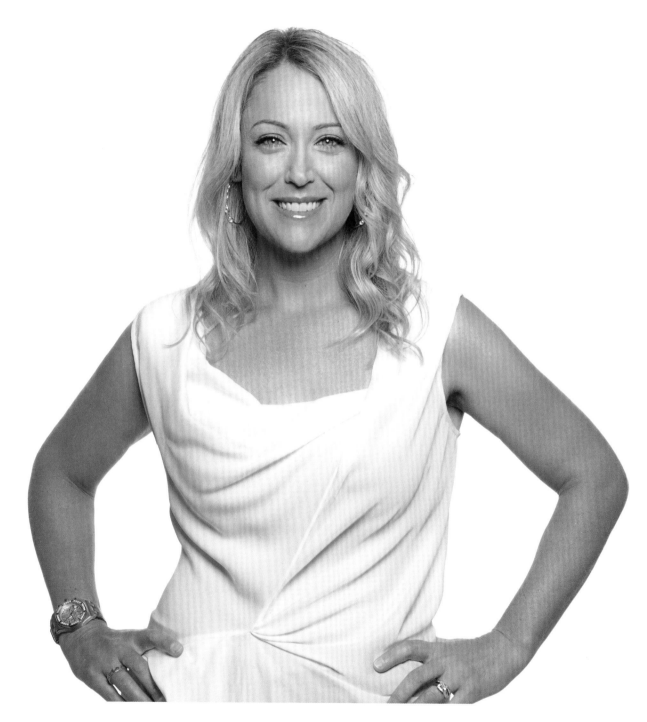

CRISTIE'S MAKEUP

To add definition to Cristie's sparkling eyes, I went with a dark charcoal powder liner for the top lash line. For blondes, charcoal rather than black is a great choice for making eyes pop without being too intense.

I want girls to know that it doesn't matter if you think you're not pretty, because you are. You just have to let the inside show on the outside.

—CRISTIE KERR

When I was thirteen I was told I would never play professional golf. I had a devastating injury running at school, and over the next few years, I kept reinjuring myself and had to have major surgery. I am proud to have overcome that and become the golfer and person that I am now.

I was very overweight as a child. In my teens I ballooned up to 180 pounds. I had a frizzy perm and glasses. I didn't feel very pretty. I overcame that when I saw my relatives getting sick and having health problems, and I didn't want to end up like them. I went to see a trainer and a nutritionist. Just with dieting and exercise, I was able to lose about seventy pounds in about two years.

There are really no words to describe the way you feel when you are at the top of your sport. It's just elation, unbelievable happiness, and exhaustion. It's all of that wrapped into one package.

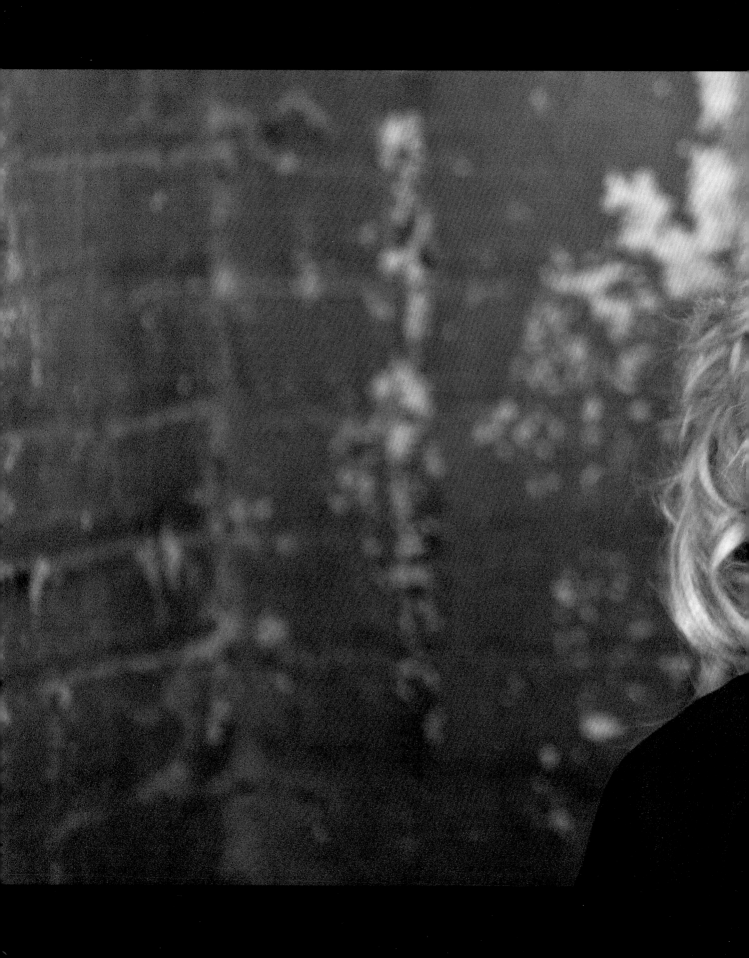

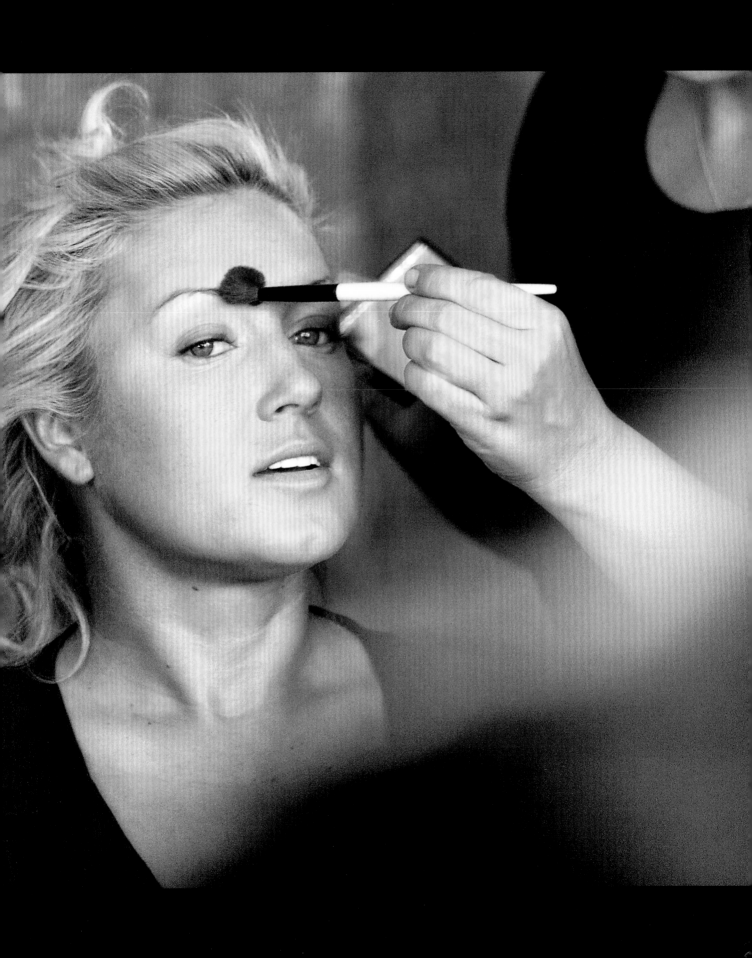

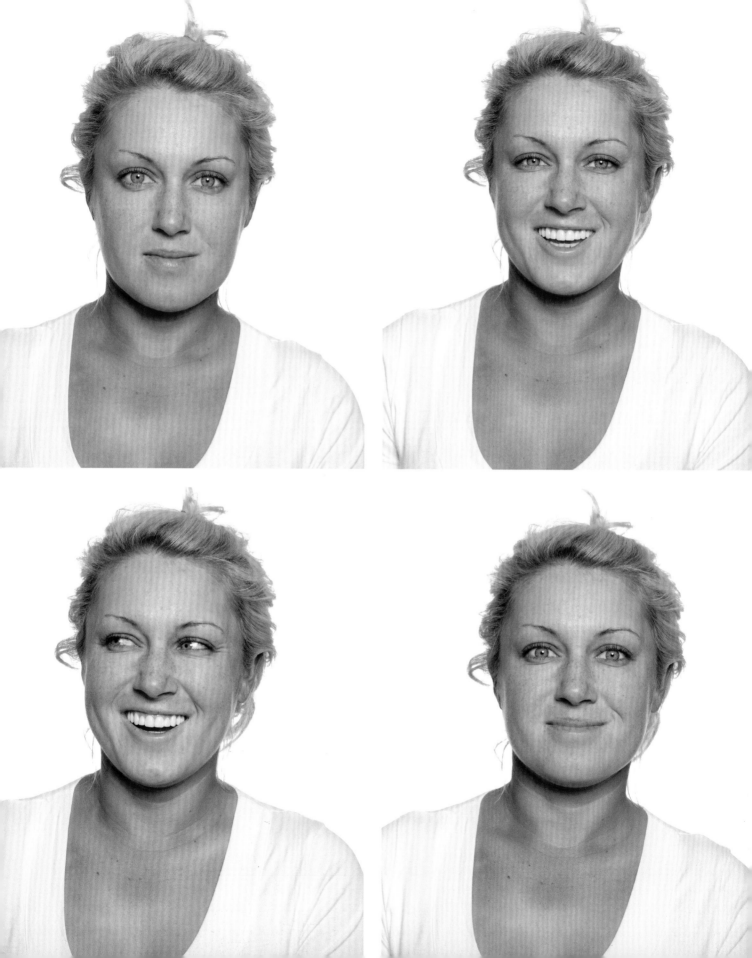

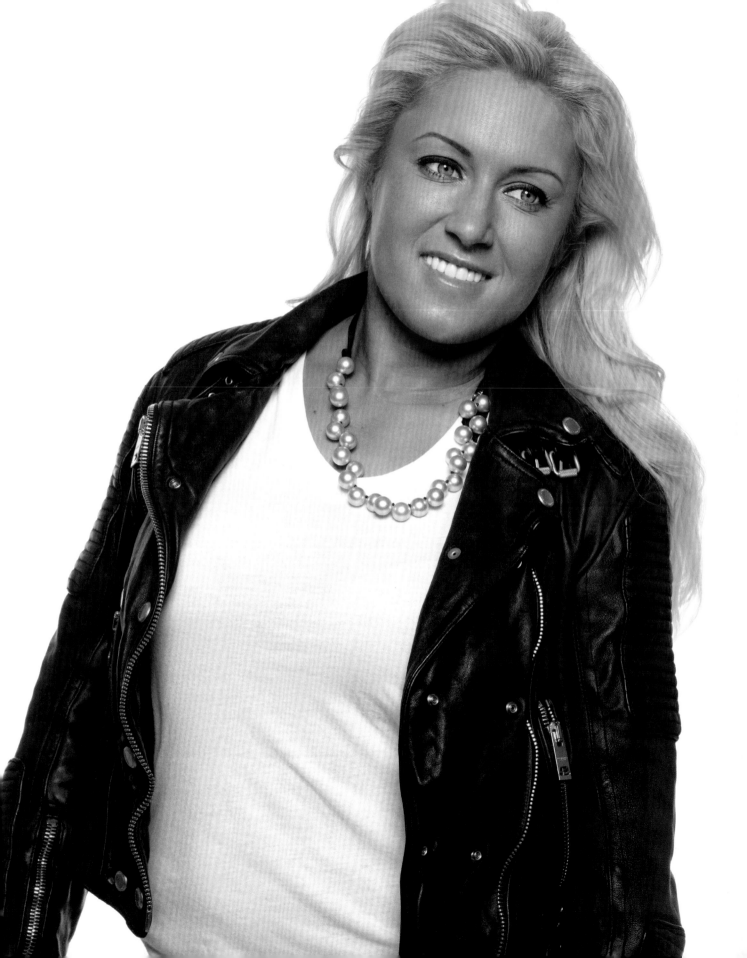

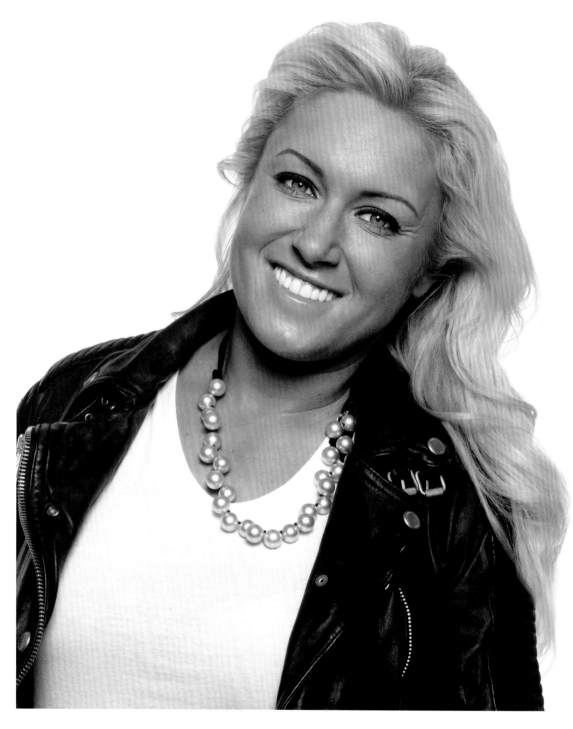

NATALIE'S MAKEUP

Natalie is very girly and loves makeup. I wanted to show how pretty she looks with more subtle makeup than she usually wears—just bronzer, blush, lip gloss, and a touch of dark brown smoky liner. Sometimes less is more. I love the juxtaposition of her strong leather jacket with the pink pearls.

The best part of my life is that I get to give back.

—NATALIE GULBIS

I played in my first LGPA event when I was fourteen. When you're that age, the whole world is in front of you and you think you can do anything. My mom and dad always inspired me to set limitless goals, and that was the perfect example.

I've had a dream life and a great professional and golf career, but the best part of my life is that I get to give back. When you finally get to the level that you can use your name and awareness for different charities, it's great. I'm involved with fifteen charities. My hope is to open up a Boys & Girls Club. I love being with kids and I love that it is a place that gives them a chance.

For years I wore a ton of makeup and tried to cover my face. I thought wearing more was better! Bobbi taught me how to take care of my skin and how to put on makeup. Bobbi has completely changed my look.

LAUREL WASSNER
&
REBECCAH WASSNER
PROFESSIONAL TRIATHLETES

The first thing you notice about Laurel and Rebeccah Wassner is that they are always smiling. They have great energy and come into a room beaming. The twin sisters have a lot to smile about these days—after battling Hodgkin's lymphoma at twenty-three, Laurel is now healthy and competing alongside her sister as a professional triathlete. At 5'3", the sisters are petite powerhouses. They are incredibly strong and lean. All it took was a little makeup and some sky-high YSL heels, and Rebeccah and Laurel went from sporty to sophisticated.

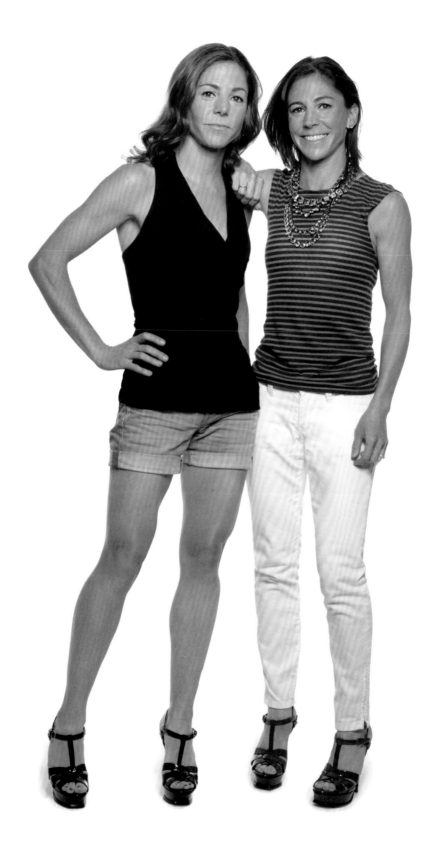

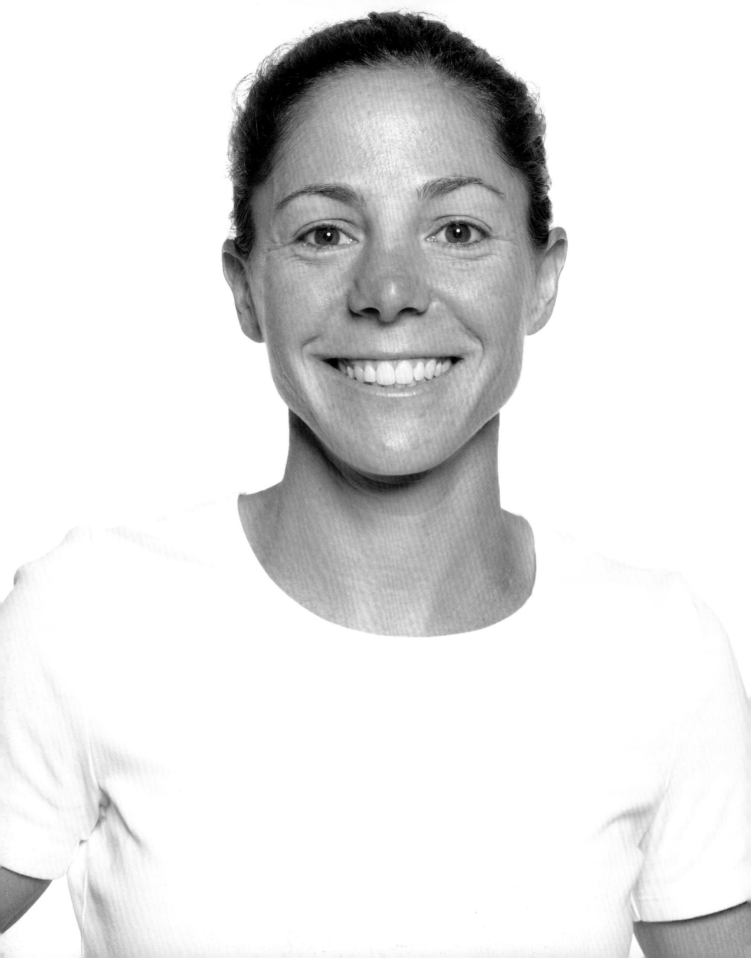

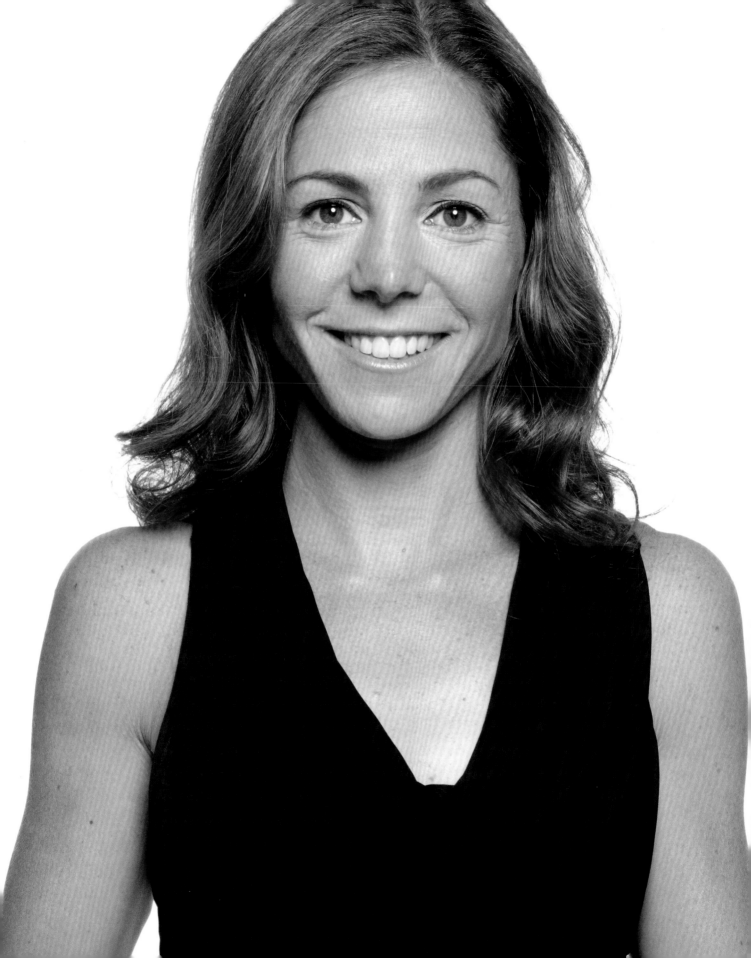

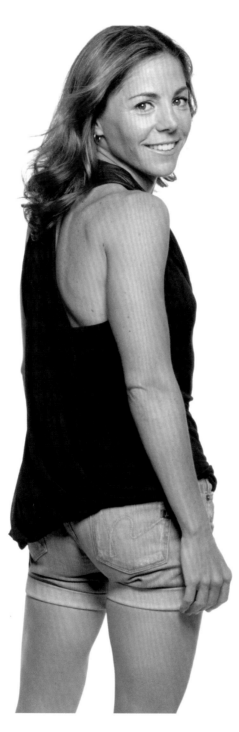

LAUREL'S MAKEUP

Laurel has the look of a healthy, fresh girl next door. I enhanced her clear eyes, freckles, and outdoorsy glow with minimal makeup—a little blush, nude eye shadows, and a brown liner.

Going through chemotherapy is something that has made me stronger.

—LAUREL WASSNER

Going through chemotherapy—hearing "you have cancer"—is something that has made me stronger. As an athlete, I draw on that strength daily. It helps me when I get out there and race because racing isn't easy either.

I'm happiest when I'm running. I smile while I am running. I just love the freedom I have. I am so lucky to be out there. There was a long time when I couldn't even run for two minutes.

I'm really proud that I got away from my desk job when it was eighty degrees outside. I just said, "I'm going to be a triathlete," and I did it without any reservations, and it worked out—fortunately! It was a risk leaving a stable job and going to a job where I might not even get paid if I didn't win. I'm really proud that I made the leap.

When I was going through chemotherapy, my sisters would take me to the Bobbi Brown counter. We would get makeovers and it was a way to feel good during a tough time.

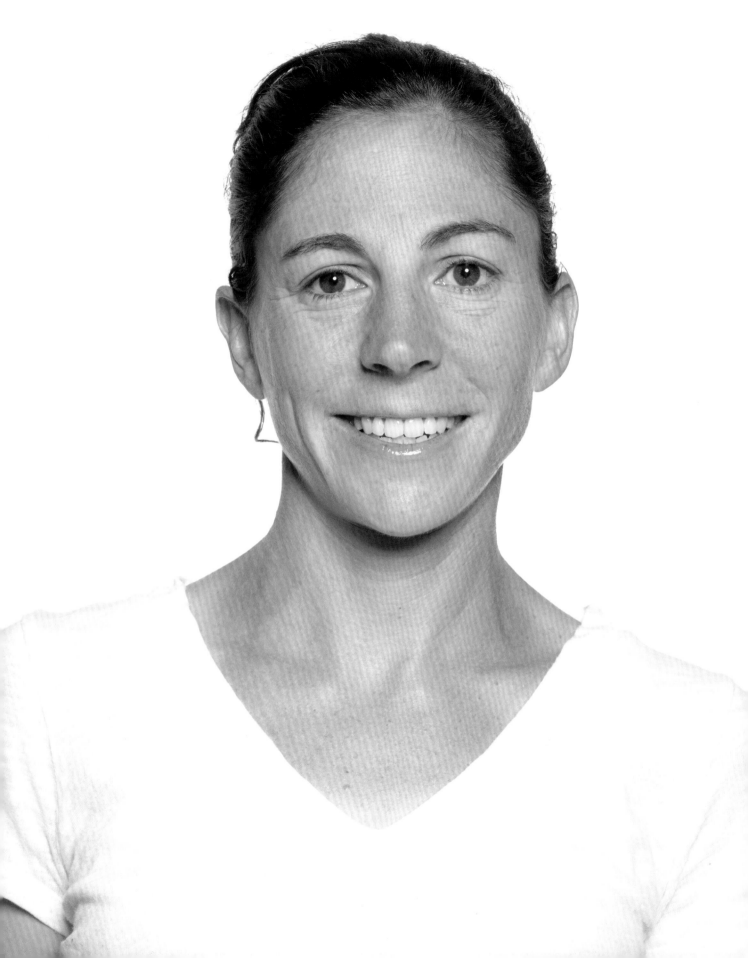

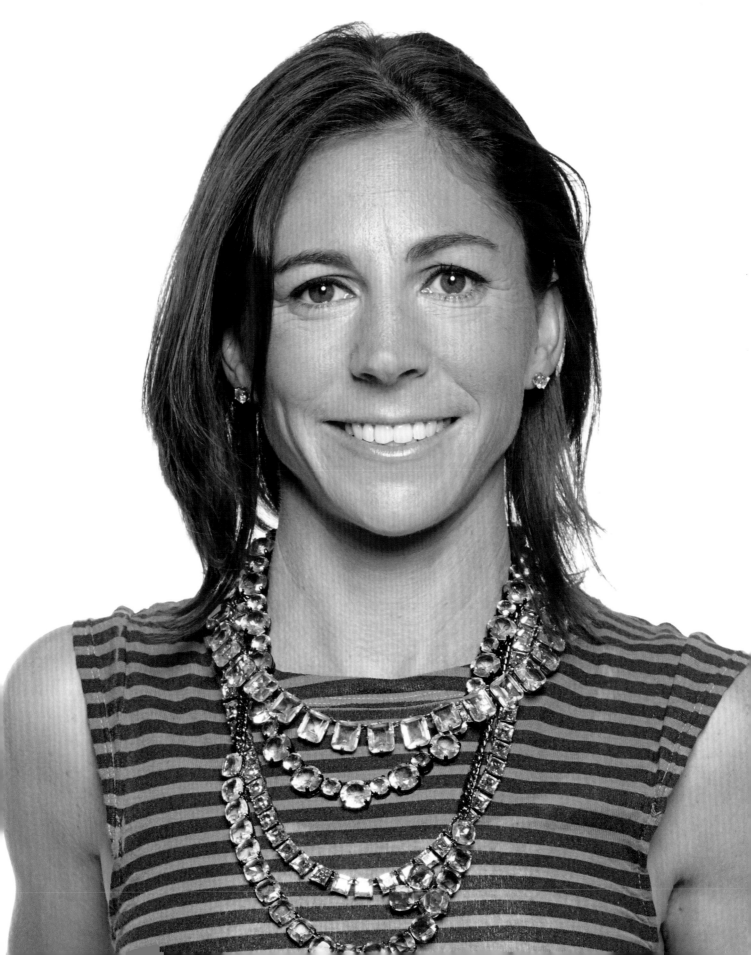

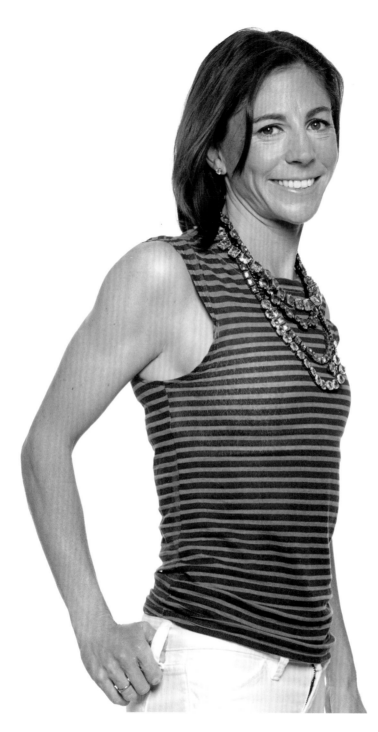

REBECCAH'S MAKEUP

Rebeccah went from looking fresh-faced to elegant with only a touch of makeup. I minimized the slight redness in her skin from being in the sun with tinted moisturizer and mineral powder. Mineral powder is a great choice for athletes because it counteracts oily skin (you just have to make sure it looks natural). Then I added a pop of blush, pink lips, and black liner for a little bit of drama.

Once I set my mind to something, nothing is going to get in my way.

—REBECCAH WASSNER

When I first started doing triathlons, I was really excited to meet this guru of the sport who had just written a book. I told him I was going to be a pro triathlete, and probably because I'm small and a lot shorter than any professional triathlete, he looked at me and kind of laughed and said, "Good luck." I walked away and thought, *Wow, this guy just brushed me off!* But I knew that I had the desire and the will and just because somebody looked at me and thought that I wasn't going to be good, it wasn't going to stop me.

Laurel's cancer made me see things differently and take advantage of every day. I was an accountant, but it really wasn't doing it for me. I knew I could be a good athlete, but I needed something to push me to try it. When I realized I could pay the bills, I said, "I'm going to try this. I have no reason not to now." So that experience probably changed both of us.

Once I set my mind to something, nothing is going to get in my way. Physically, I'm on the smaller side, but most of my strength comes from within.

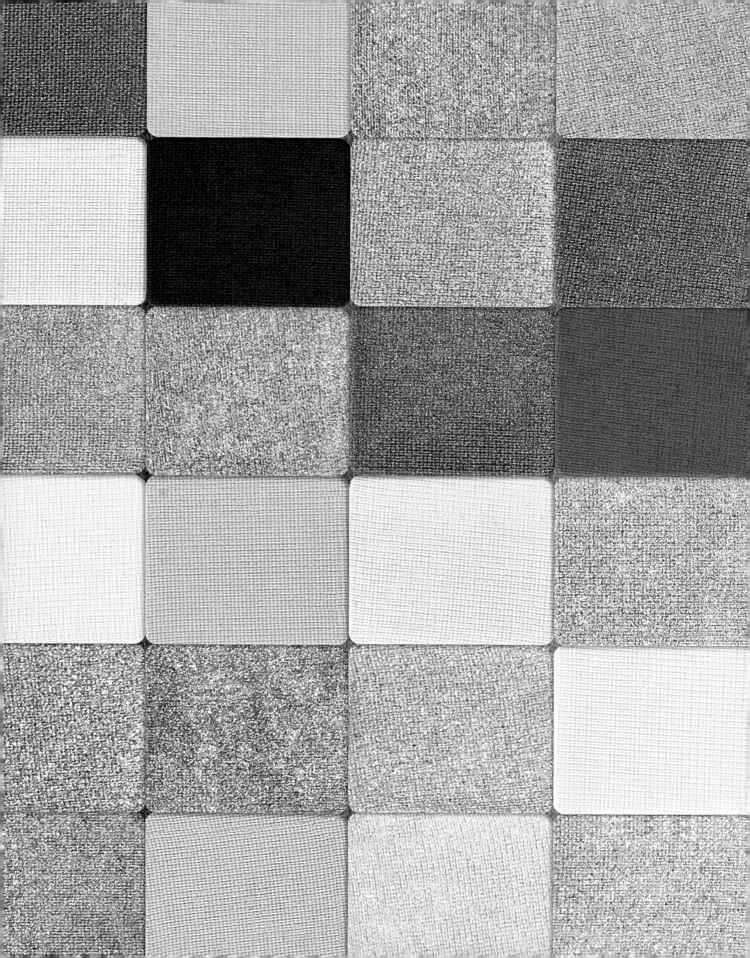

04

PRETTY CLASSIC

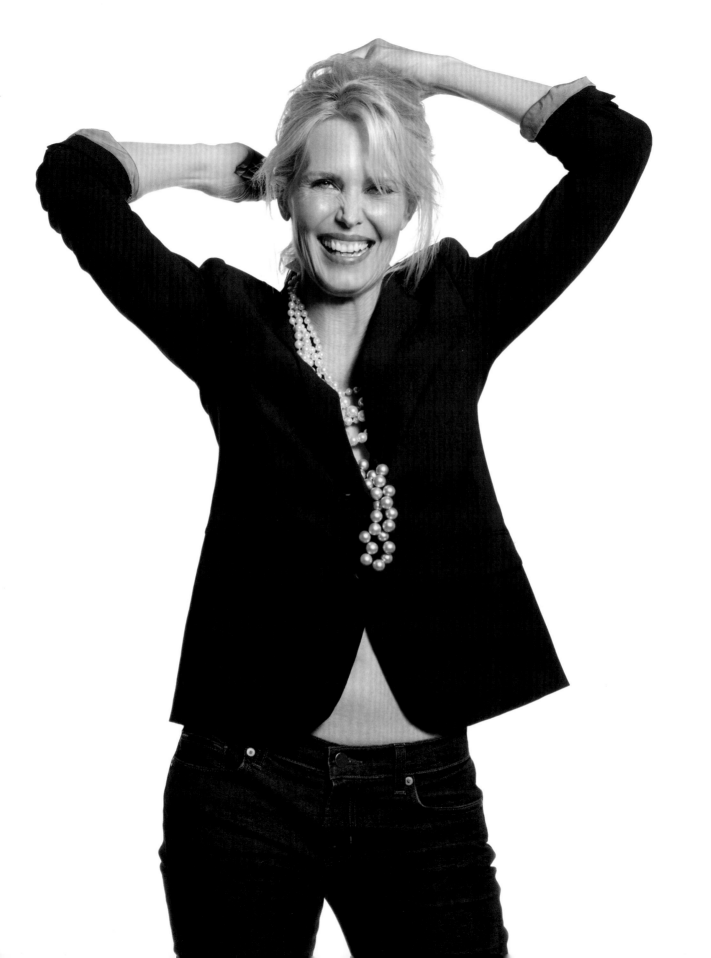

PRETTY CLASSIC

Pretty Classic women epitomize timeless style. They wear jewelry that once belonged to their mothers (and they plan to pass it down to their daughters). They carry on the tradition of reading the same bedtime stories to their children that their grandparents read to them. Having good manners and writing thank-you notes—not emails—is simply a part of who they are. Appreciating the past, however, doesn't mean that they don't love fashion and high style. Think of the stunning iconic supermodel Carmen, who is both über-classic and very chic. The amazing Ralph Lauren reinvented the classic look with gorgeous clothes that never go out of style. Ralph's muse and beautiful wife, Ricky, is a perfect example of the Pretty Classic woman.

I love the classic look. Blue jeans, a great blazer, and pink pearl earrings are my staples. I collect and wear Ted Muehling's modernized pearls. And I adore the simplicity of Helen Ficalora's charm necklaces—I wear a peace sign and the first initials of my three sons on a gold beaded chain daily. I'm also a fan of monograms (I even have monogrammed clogs). My many monogrammed L.L. Bean bags help organize my life. I have them labeled *Work, Beach, Home,* and *Dogs,* and a big one for donations says *Give.*

I admire women who are Pretty Classic, because they are consistent with not only their style, but also with everything. They are trustworthy, solid, and dependable—qualities I strive for myself.

CLASSIC BEAUTY

The secrets behind polished makeup

DAY

SKIN

A classic look starts with perfect, even skin, which you can achieve by using the correct foundation formula for your skin type. Whether the foundation is matte, sheer, or richly moisturizing, you want it to eliminate redness and create the appearance of even skin.

CHEEKS

You'll need two blushes. Your basic blush should be the color your cheeks turn when you exercise. Top that with a pop of a brighter color applied to the apples of the cheeks. Apply a bit of rich moisturizer on top of the blush for an extra glow.

EYES

To create a classic eye, you'll need three basic eye shadows: light, medium, and dark. Start by brushing the lightest shade all over the lid with a full eye shadow brush. Then apply the medium shade from the lash line to just above the crease. Finish by lining the top lash line with the darkest shadow using either a damp or dry eyeliner brush. To give your eyes a finishing touch, apply a couple of coats of very black mascara. When it is almost dry, bend your lashes up with your finger. This is an easy way to give your lashes some extra curl.

For polished brows, start by working with a professional to create the ideal shape for your face (you can then keep up the shape on your own with tweezers). Fill in your brow using a brow pencil or a slanted brush and shadow. The shade should match your hair color.

LIPS

A classic lip is pretty and feminine. To get the look, choose a lip color that is a little bit brighter than your regular lip—whether that is rose, pink, or peach. For added definition, use a pencil in the same color as your lip color.

HAIR

Classic hair is polished and well maintained. Hair is always perfectly cut and colored with no lapses between appointments that might result in roots showing or a slightly imperfect 'do. The shape of the hair is never trendy, but timeless—chic bobs, crisp bangs, and clean layers set the tone.

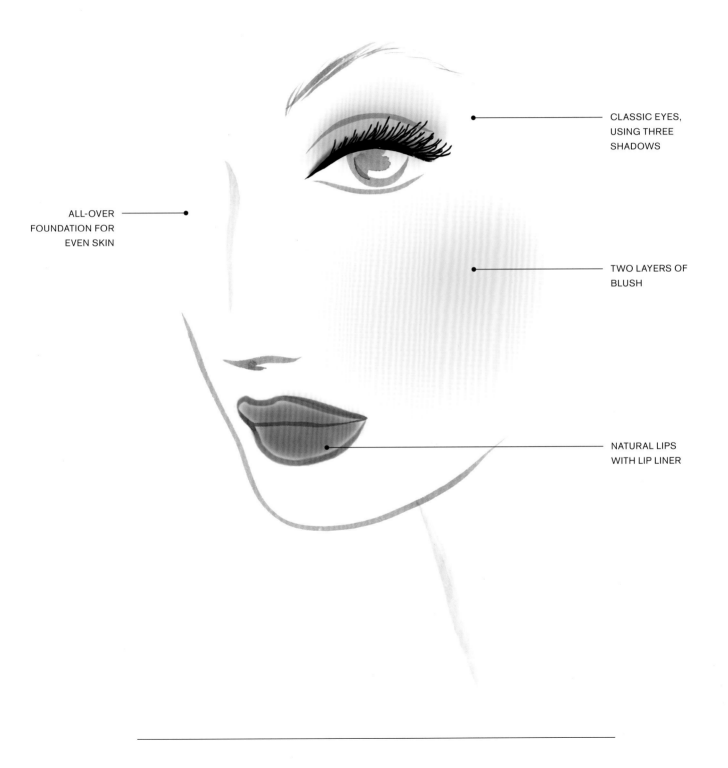

CLASSIC EYES,
USING THREE
SHADOWS

ALL-OVER
FOUNDATION FOR
EVEN SKIN

TWO LAYERS OF
BLUSH

NATURAL LIPS
WITH LIP LINER

CLASSIC BEAUTY

Go a little brighter

———

EVENING

SKIN

For night you want a bit more coverage. Add touches of your daytime foundation along with concealer to areas where your makeup has faded. Another option is to use a very natural powder foundation formula that will stay on longer and provide additional coverage and polish.

CHEEKS

Add texture on top of the two-blush combination you use for day. A powder shimmer or a liquid highlighter applied to the top of the cheekbone, a little higher than where you normally apply blush, will catch the light beautifully.

EYES

To open up the eyes, line them all the way around with a black or caviar liner. Layer on two to three coats of mascara—a soft grey or slate adds depth without being too harsh. A touch of highlight shadow just underneath the brow bone completes the look.

LIPS

Go for a shade that is brighter than your daytime color. Anything pale will make you look washed out. Brighter, matte color is timeless.

HAIR

A blowout always gives your hair a shiny and polished finish and complements a beautiful cut and color.

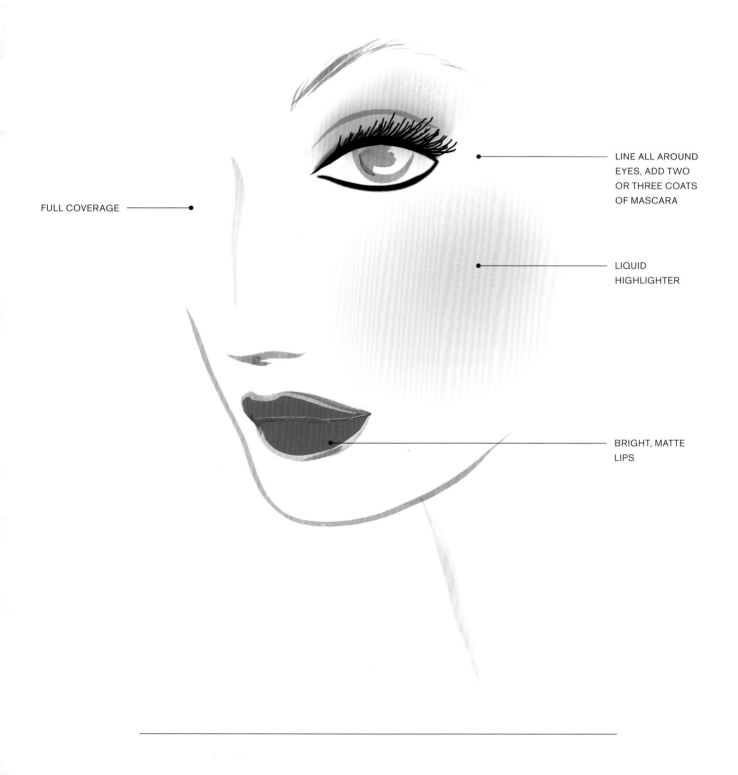

FULL COVERAGE

LINE ALL AROUND
EYES, ADD TWO
OR THREE COATS
OF MASCARA

LIQUID
HIGHLIGHTER

BRIGHT, MATTE
LIPS

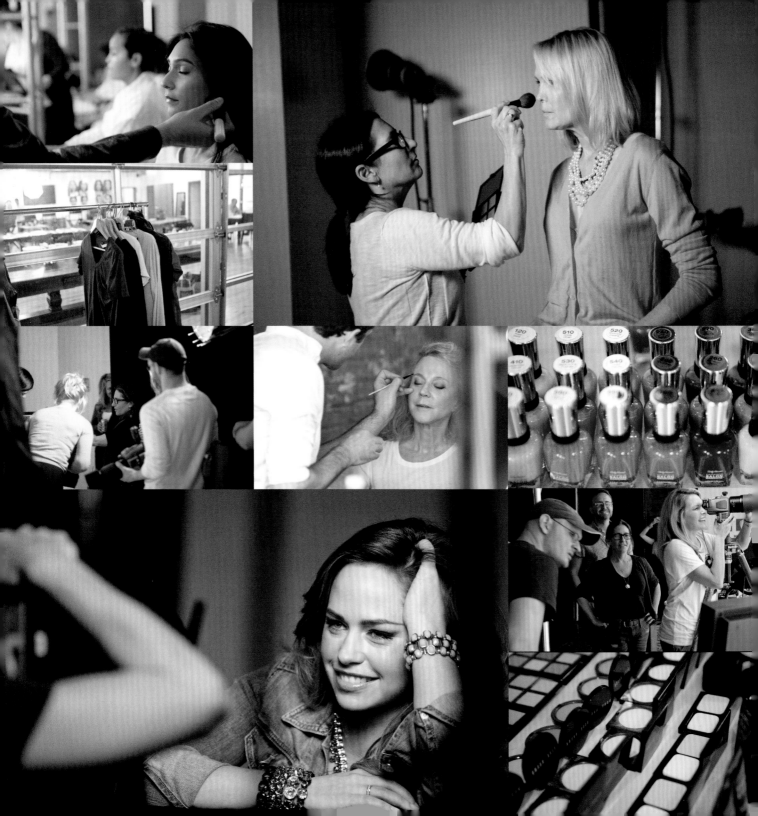

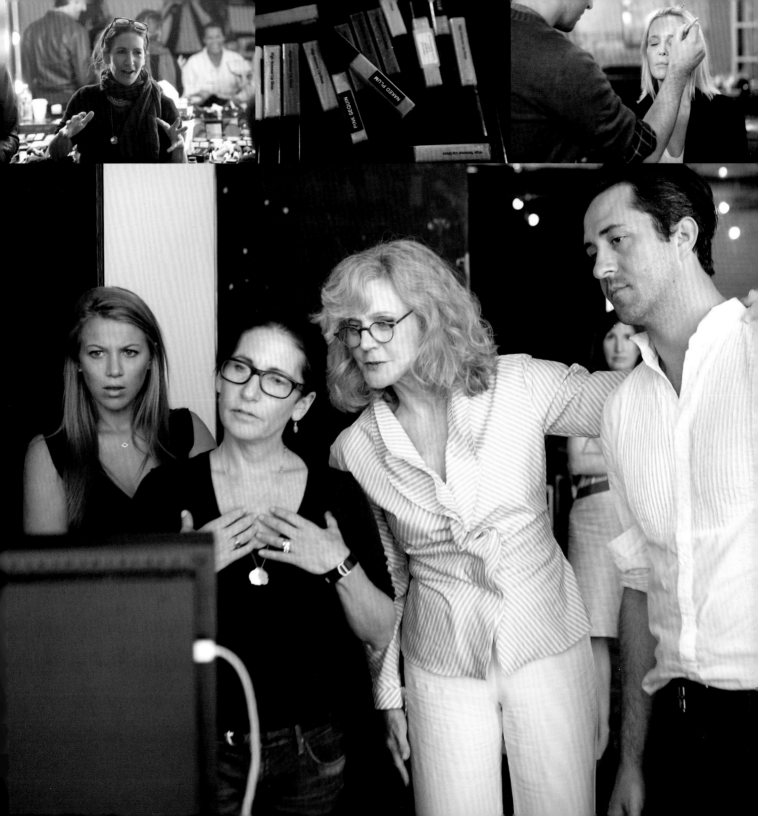

NANCY DONAHUE
BEAUTY INDUSTRY ENTREPRENEUR

———

Years before I met Nancy, I was a fan. She graced the covers of *Mademoiselle*, *Glamour*, and *Vogue* and was always classically stunning. I've gotten to know Nancy, and she is real, earthy, and as beautiful on the inside as she is on the outside. Nancy has evolved from cover girl to yoga teacher to entrepreneur and continues to look amazing and be graceful along the way.

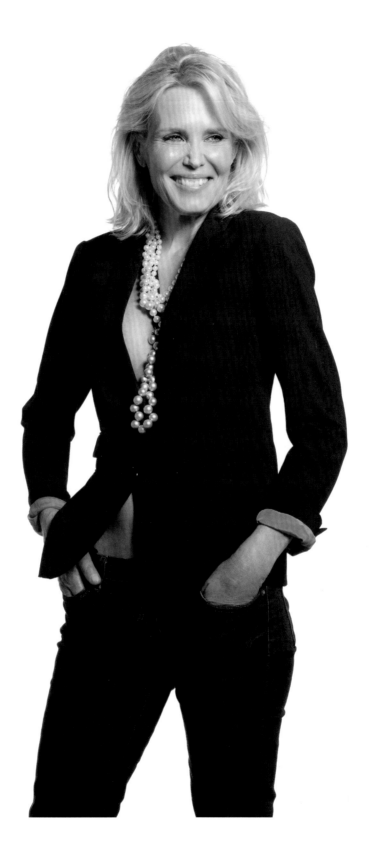

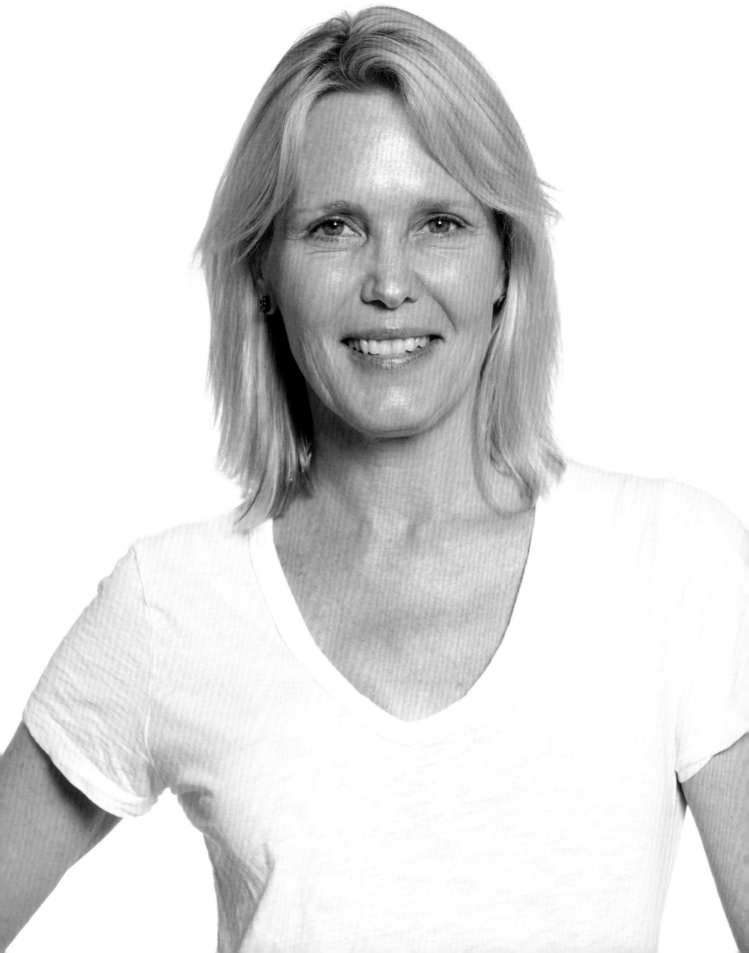

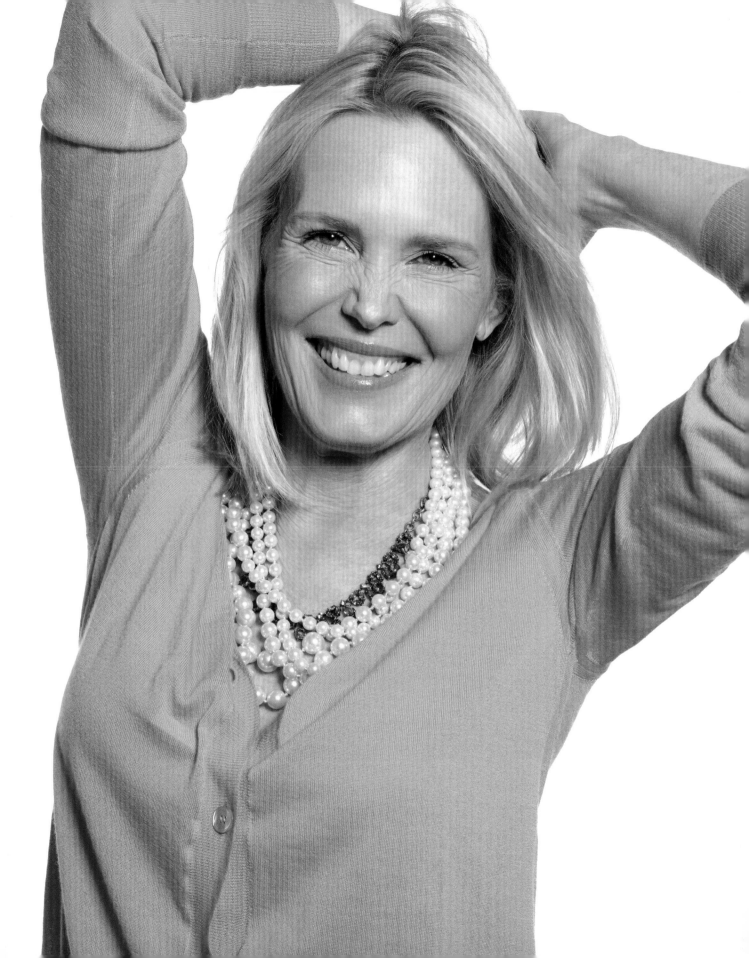

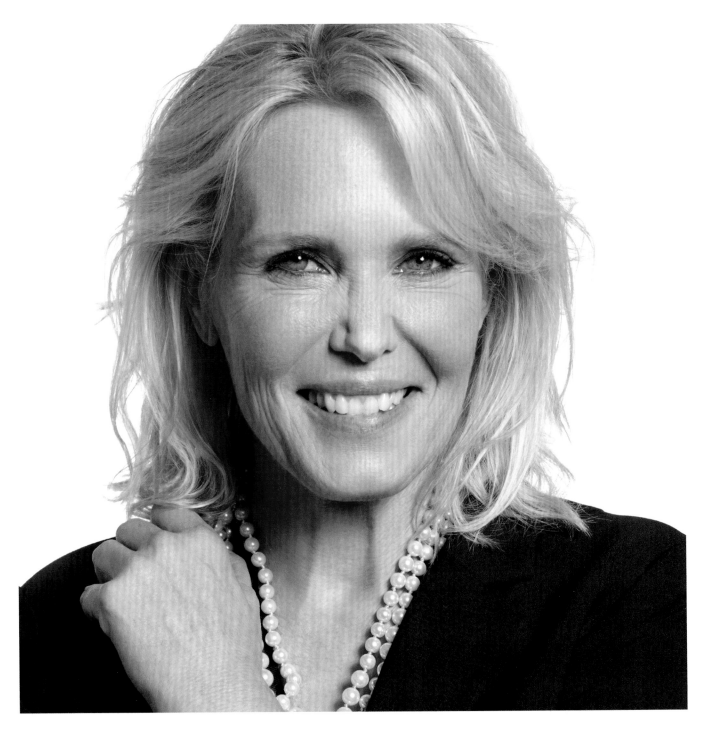

NANCY'S MAKEUP

On blondes, light brows and eyelashes tend to disappear, so I gave Nancy more definition with a medium ash beige shadow on her brows, a color that is in the same tone as her hair. An indigo gel liner instantly brings out her eyes. On her cheeks and lips, shades of pink that are not too bright and not too wimpy add just the right amount of softness. Nancy's face comes alive with makeup.

My parents gave me the best life advice. Work hard and be nice!

—NANCY DONAHUE

Fitness transformed my life. I became a triathlete, marathoner, yoga teacher, Pilates teacher, and a personal trainer. I just thought, *This is where my place is.*

My motto is "The glass is always half full." I'm super positive. I never go the down route. My glass is never empty, or even half empty, ever!

Concealer and bronzer are my two favorite things. I can't live without them.

Exercise, eating good food, feeling a lot of love, being positive, and having a good outlook on life all make me feel pretty.

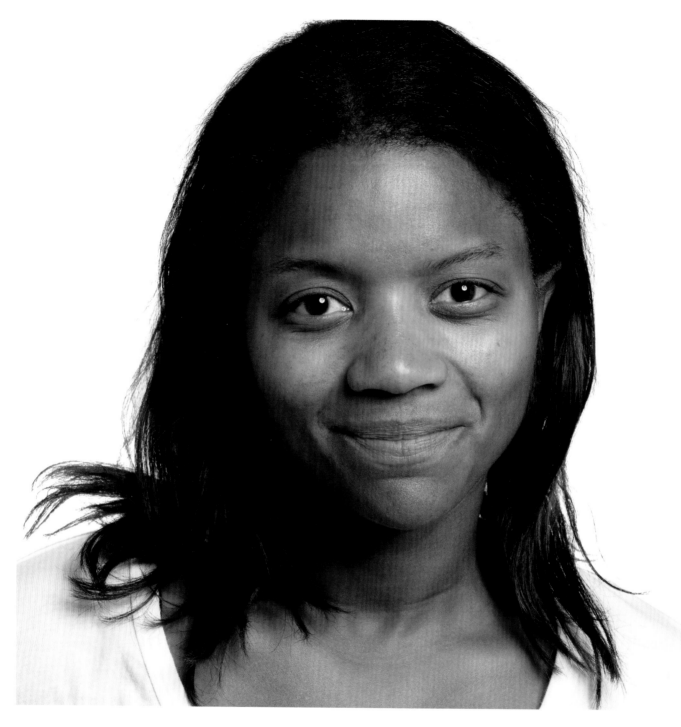

JACQUIE ANTINORO MOTHER

My favorite never-fail makeup trick is eyeliner.

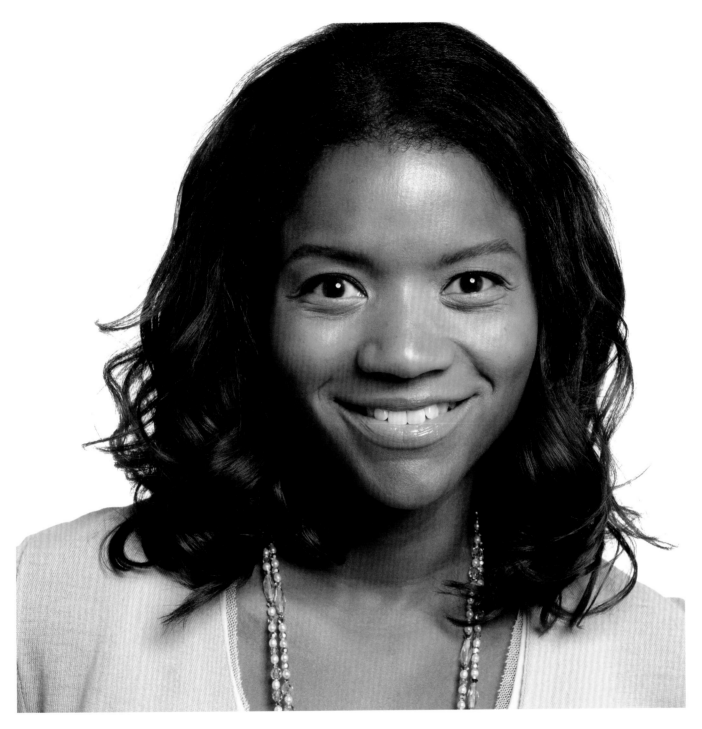

JACQUIE'S MAKEUP

A peach tone corrector and honey-colored concealer counteract undereye darkness and bring a terrific brightness to Jacquie's face. We relied on sheer lip gloss and an apricot blush to give her gorgeous face a little glow.

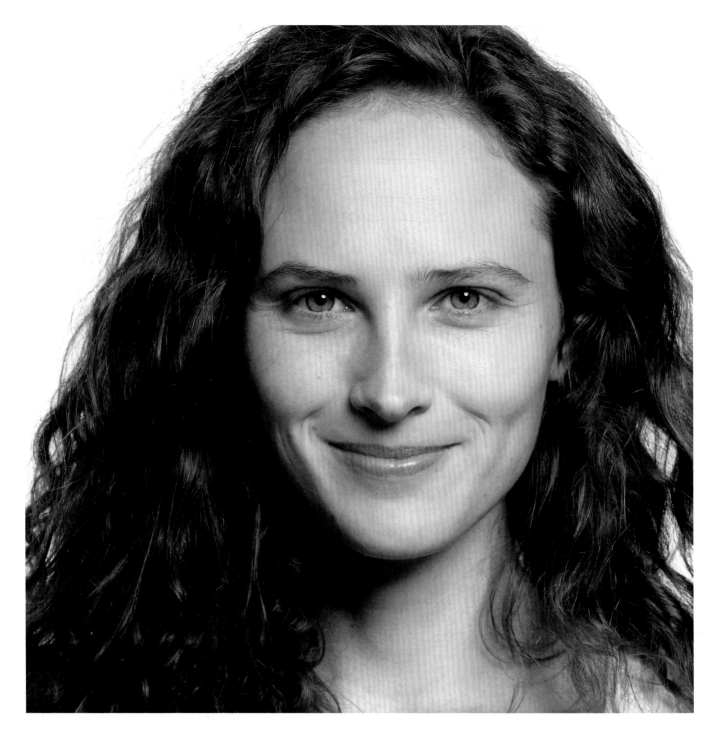

SASKIA MILLER
ACTRESS, COMMUNICATIONS STRATEGIST, WRITER

The best compliment I ever received is that my intelligence makes me attractive and beautiful.

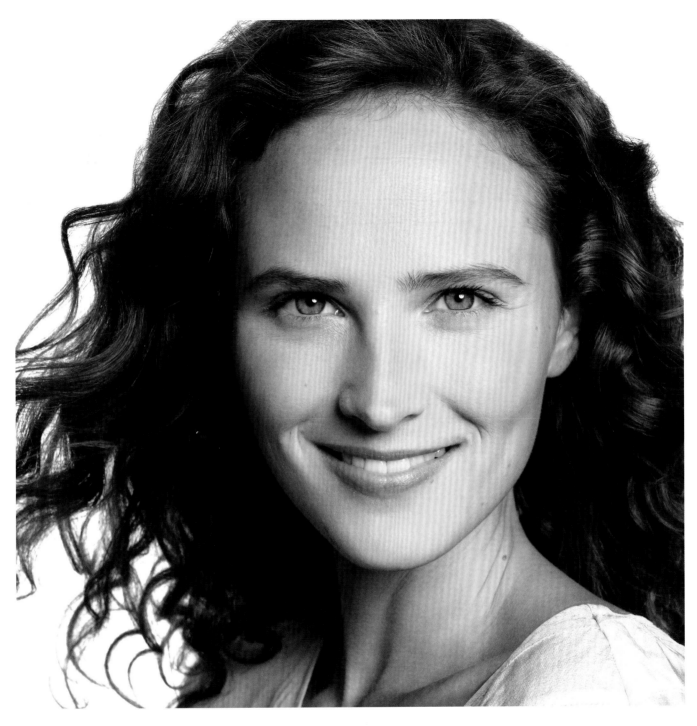

SASKIA'S MAKEUP

Saskia has beautiful bluish-green eyes that stand out against her dark brown hair. Concealer combined with a very light touch of gray eye shadow on the lids, black liner, and mascara illuminate her eyes even more.

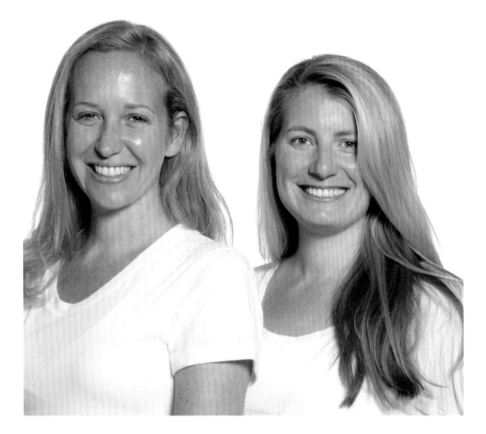

ALEXANDRA WILSON
&
ALEXIS MAYBANK
COFOUNDERS, GILT GROUPE

Cofounders of the revolutionary online shopping site Gilt Groupe, best friends Alexandra and Alexis met at Harvard Business School. After Alexis helped launch eBay and Alexandra worked her retailing magic at Bulgari, they teamed up with the idea to bring private New York sample sales to the masses. Gilt now sells everything from vacations to gourmet food. Alexandra and Alexis are an example of how working with your best friend can make your friendship stronger (in the beginning they vowed never to let their professional relationship take over the friendship). They are also models for how turning your passion into a business can be a recipe for success.

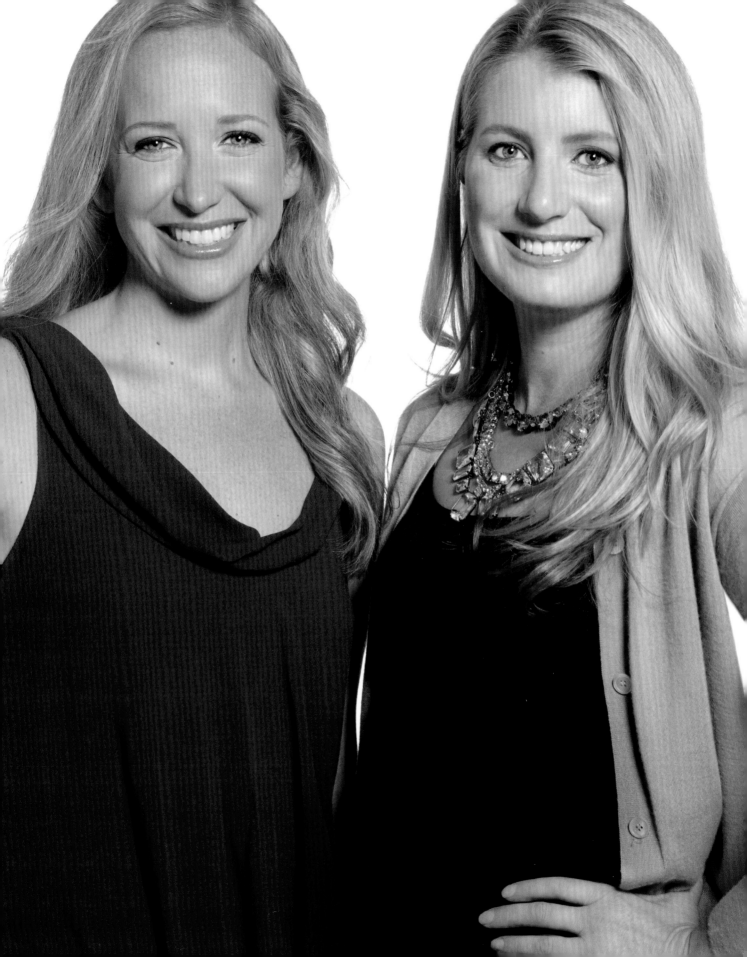

You only live once.

—ALEXANDRA WILSON

I think it's important to, every so often, reflect on what it is that you're looking for, what it is that makes you happy, and who makes you happy. And to keep that in your mind as you live your day-to-day life, because it's easy to lose sight of what's most important.

I wish I knew when I was eighteen that it is possible to make a successful career out of what you really love and what comes naturally. I didn't realize I could make a career out of fashion and shopping and a love of clothes and design.

As a child growing up in New York City, I was different from a lot of my friends. I'm half Cuban, I'm half Jewish, my hair is sort of strawberry blonde, and these were all things that made me different. I think when you're a kid, you so badly want to blend in and be just like your peers, and over time you realize that being unique is actually an asset and is what makes you special.

There's something really special about working with and learning from a friend. It is not about ego; it's about sharing and teaching the other person what you know a lot about.

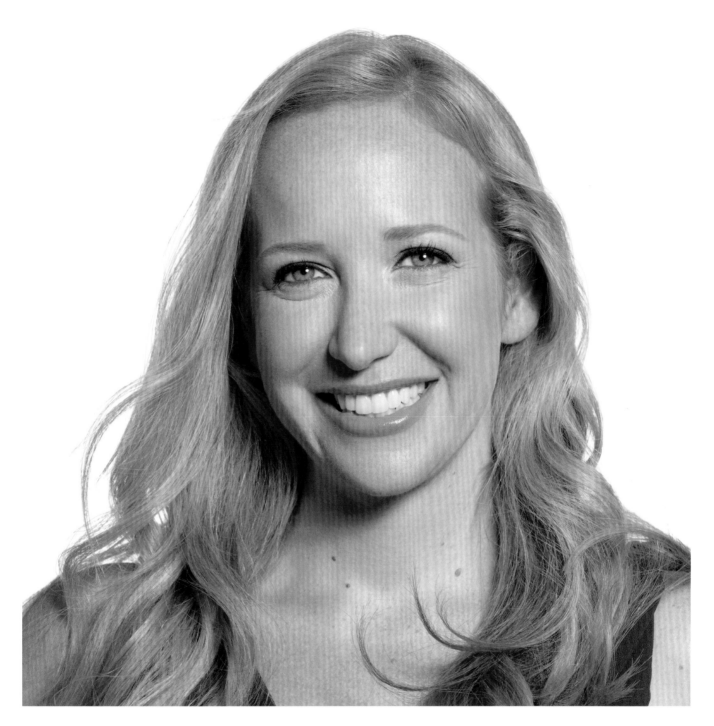

ALEXANDRA'S MAKEUP

For strawberry blondes like Alexandra, a medium brown bronzer placed where the sun naturally hits the skin, paired with a pop of a light pink illuminating bronzer on cheeks, highlights their natural glow.

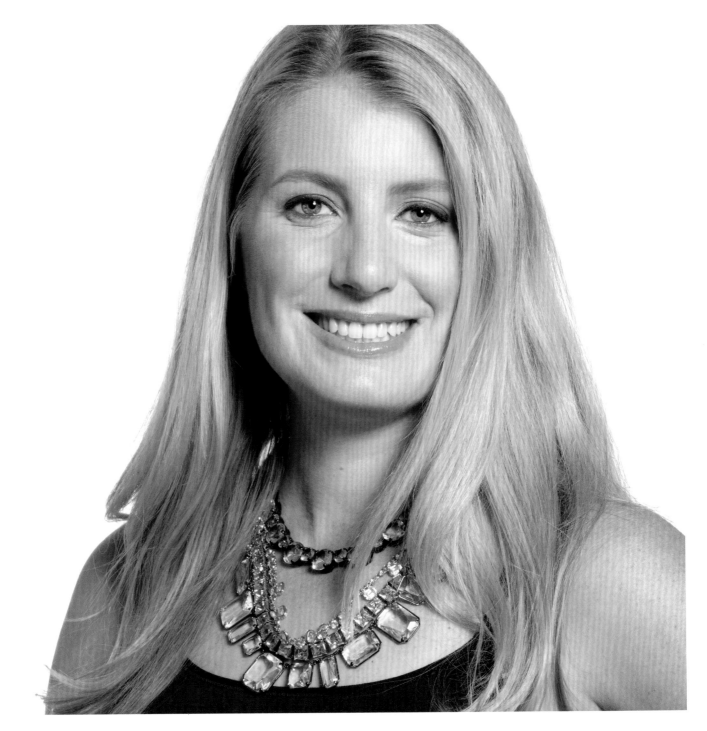

ALEXIS'S MAKEUP

For women with fair skin and blonde hair like Alexis, makeup really helps to bring out their features, especially their eyes. We brought out Alexis's gorgeous eyes with a cool eye shadow palette of pinkish white, silvery brown, and mauve shimmer, along with black mascara, and a rich beige shadow on her brows. We lined her eyes with a black gel liner and softened the look by smudging a silvery-gray shadow on top. With dusty-pink lips and cheeks, Alexis's look is fun and sophisticated.

Confidence in what I'm doing, what I can do, and what I have done makes me feel powerful.

—ALEXIS MAYBANK

In my early twenties, I thought that there were models of success, meaning that you had to act a certain way and dress a certain way in a business environment. I received very good advice, actually from a man, to develop my own personal style. You have to be very comfortable in order to be confident. So that means presenting yourself, speaking, and thinking in ways that are very personal to you and your own style. The more you are true to yourself—and don't force yourself into a mold—the more confident you'll feel day in and day out.

I'm proudest of starting a family and following, from a career perspective, ideas that I was very passionate about.

Success is never a straight line; you're always going to go left and right, and you need to be able to get back on course quickly and never dwell too long on unanticipated turns.

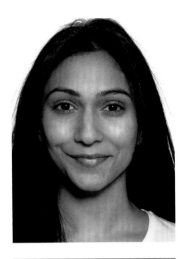

PERIVUSH SHAHZAD
PURCHASING MANAGER

My motto is "Dance like no one is watching."

PERIVUSH'S MAKEUP—DAY

To spotlight Perivush's stunning eyes, I used an off-white shadow as a base with a medium purple metallic cream shadow on the lids. For definition, I relied on a black gel liner. A golden bronzer paired with a peony blush adds enough color that I decided to keep her lips bare.

PERIVUSH'S MAKEUP—NIGHT

Taking Perivush from day to night was simple. I brought extra depth to her eyes with an ashy plum-brown shadow in the crease. For a sophisticated burst of color, I painted Perivush's full lips in a chocolate-berry lip color.

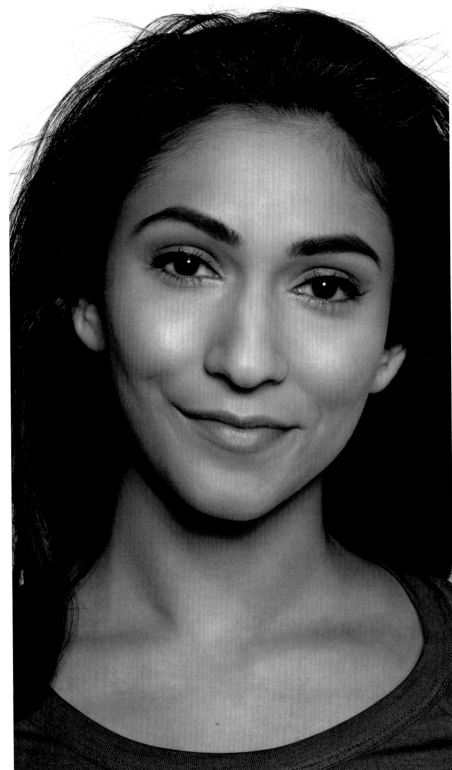

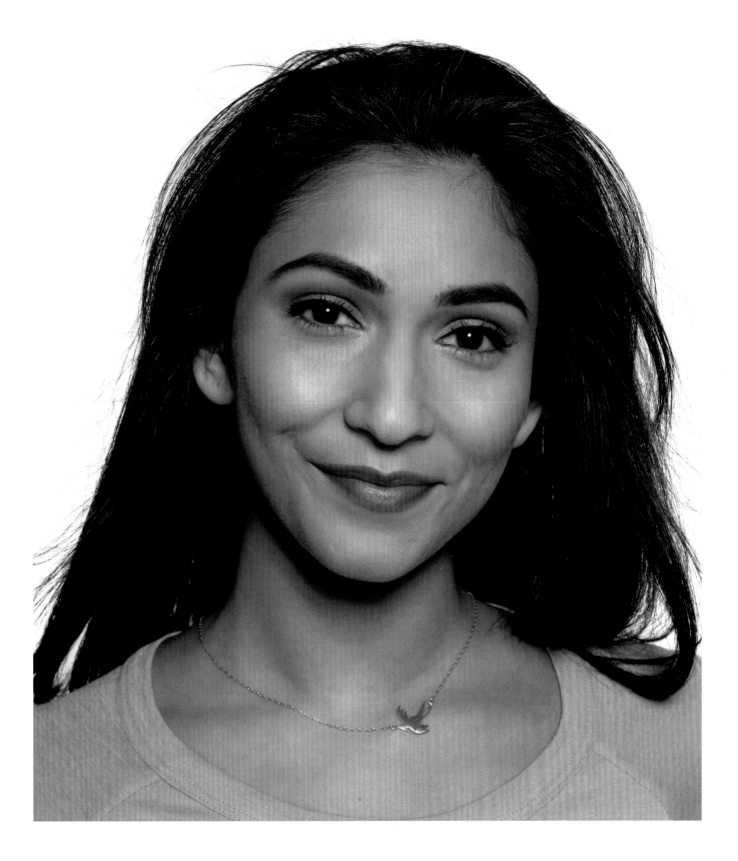

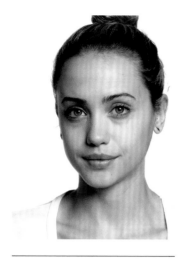

LAUREL PANTIN
BEAUTY EDITOR

My biggest indulgences are trashy novels, bad television, and dresses!

LAUREL'S MAKEUP

Laurel has great brows naturally, but enhancing them gives her a confident, flirty look. I started at the inner corner of her brow and applied a light brown shadow using a stiff angled brow brush. An ivory shadow all over the eyelid, a brownish-black gel liner, and a few coats of black mascara, paired with a soft red lip, and Laurel's ready for anything.

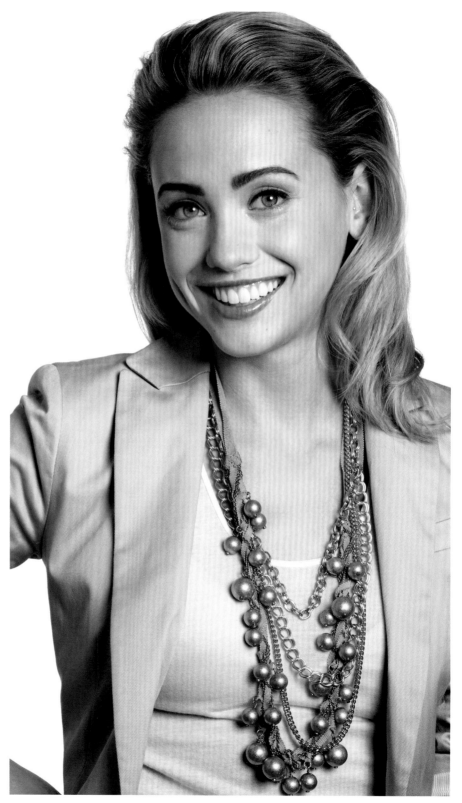

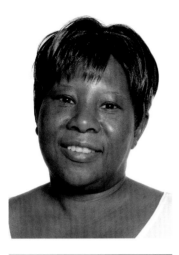

DENISE JOHNSON
HOME HEALTH AIDE,
STUDENT

My long, lean legs have been known to catch some serious attention and so has my bright, healthy mind.

DENISE'S MAKEUP

On Denise, I used a foundation brush to spot-apply a foundation stick where needed. A cranberry blush is a good choice for women with dark skin, because it is deep and bright at the same time. The color beautifully enhances Denise's terrific smile. For the most natural look, women should smile while applying their blush, placing the color right on the apples of their cheeks and blending up toward the hairline and then down to soften any visible edges.

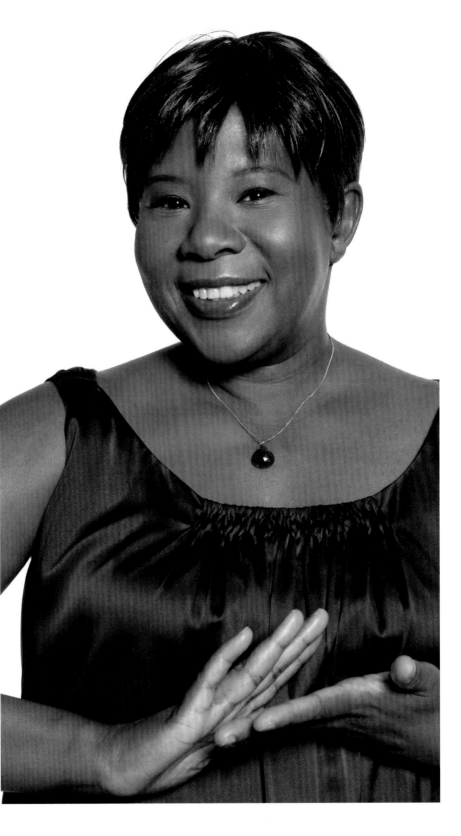

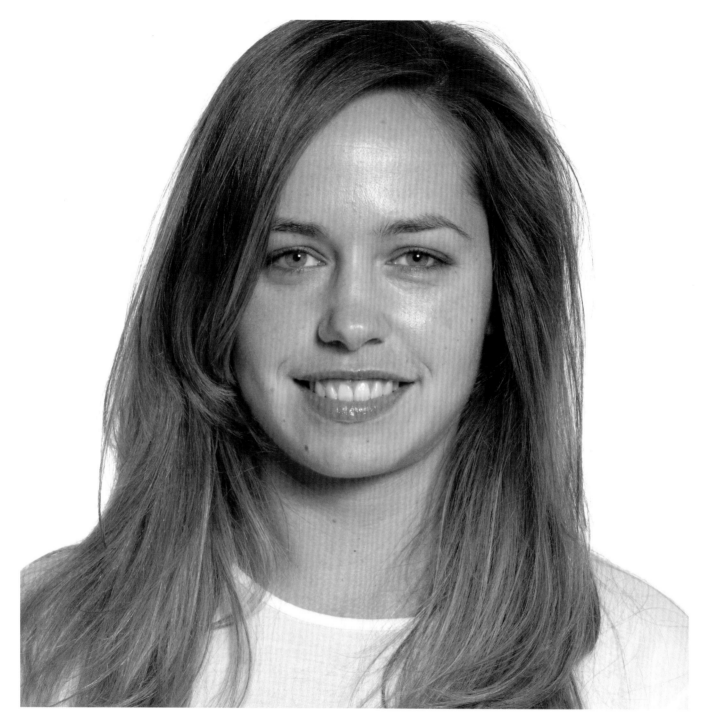

HANNAH MARTIN MAKEUP ARTIST

The best thing about my job is people and making them feel better about themselves. There is nothing better than when a woman gets off the chair and skips away. People can come in downbeat or with no confidence, and with just a little time and a bit of makeup, they leave on cloud nine.

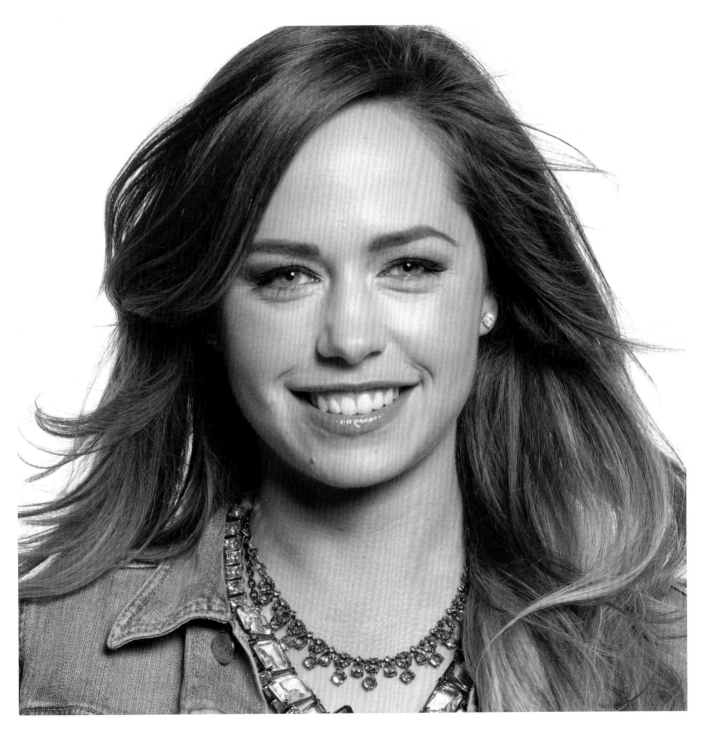

HANNAH'S MAKEUP

To bring out Hannah's eyes, we smudged a soft brown pencil on her top lash line and a slate shadow applied with a flat eyeliner brush on her lower lash line. Finishing with several coats of mascara is a sexy, but still classic, way to do a smoky eye.

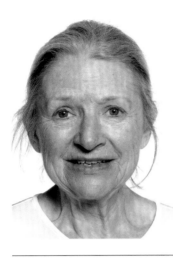

JO-ANN HOWE
RETIRED COLLEGE
ADMINISTRATOR

Reading the book Little Women *by Louisa May Alcott when I was fourteen inspired my choice of a husband and how I wanted to live our life together.*

For most of my career, I spent the majority of my time at a desk, but I tend to flourish outside, in a garden, soaking up the sun's rays (while wearing ample amounts of sunscreen, of course), without a care in the world.

JO-ANN'S MAKEUP

We focused on giving Jo-Ann an elegant yet modern look that highlights her eyes and complements her coloring. A tinted moisturizing balm hydrated her skin while offering a dewy light finish—a great choice if you have dry skin. A touch-up stick eliminated redness. I applied a rich, moisturizing eye cream to soften fine lines followed by corrector and concealer. Navy shadow applied with an eyeliner brush was a sophisticated choice that brought out her blue eyes. Bright pink lips pop against Jo-Ann's chic gray bob.

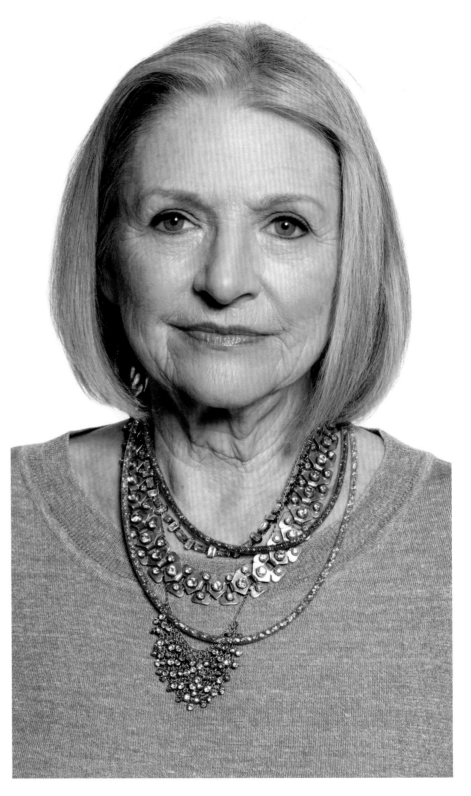

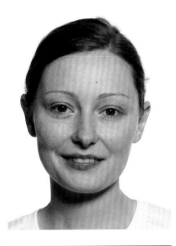

ALEXANDRA BRAZIER
VIDEO EDITOR/ PRODUCER FOR NEW MEDIA

I was really tall as a kid. I felt awkward and uncool. Being taller than every kid in school made me feel weird, not pretty. I got over it when I started to find clothes that fit well and made friends that appreciated me for my quirkiness.

ALEXANDRA'S MAKEUP

Freckles add so much personality to a face; I never cover them up. To even out Alexandra's skin while letting her gorgeous freckles shine through, I relied on a tinted moisturizer that provides sheer, lightweight coverage. For flushed cheeks that complement her porcelain skin and stunning red hair, I used an illuminating pink-coral bronzer.

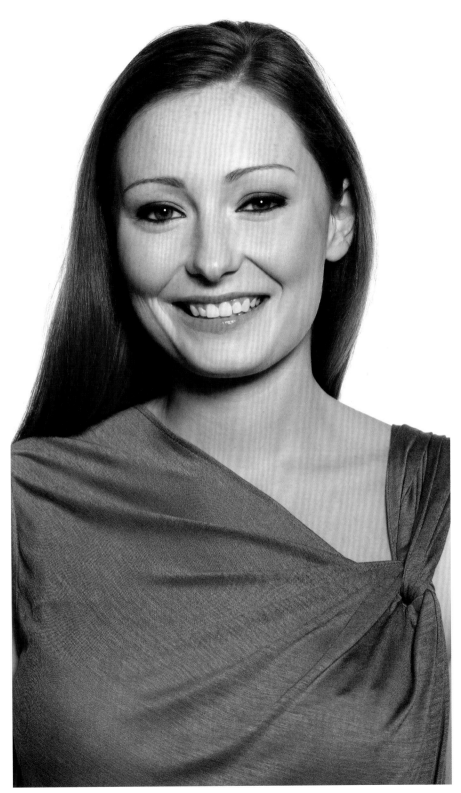

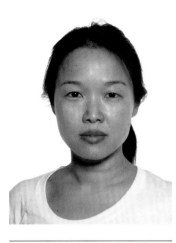

ANNE GIMM NAUGHTON
MOTHER, LAWYER, WRITER

My greatest achievement has been helping my older son become his best self. He has a developmental disability and he has had his ups and downs. I've learned so much from being his mother: what it means to grow and love a child, how to constantly engage boundaries while shaping possibilities, how a serious setback can also be the greatest gift.

ANNE'S MAKEUP— DAY

To create classic, attention-grabbing eyes, I drew a line of black gel liner on Anne's upper lash line wide enough so you can see the sweep of liner when she opens her eyes. To give her cheeks a pretty glow, I layered pink pot rouge with balm on top. Rich rose lipstick applied with a brush is a gorgeous finishing touch.

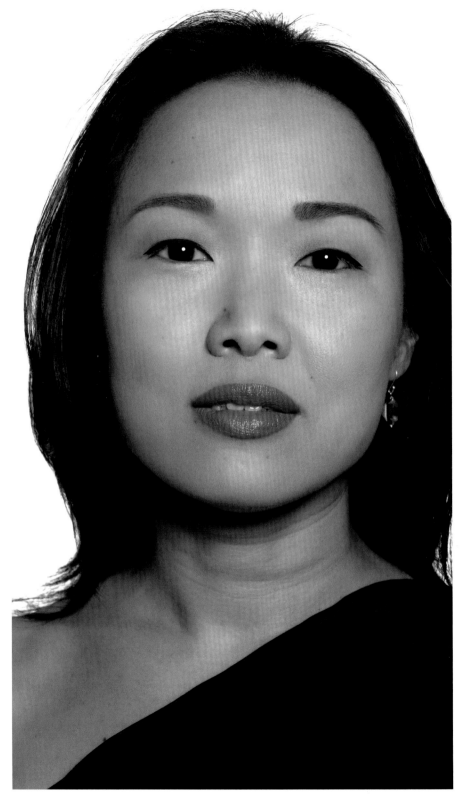

ANNE'S MAKEUP—NIGHT

To give Anne an elegantly sexy evening look, I added a platinum shimmer cream shadow on her lids and thickened and extended her eyeliner. A burst of a brighter blush with rose gloss on top of her lipstick, and she's ready to go.

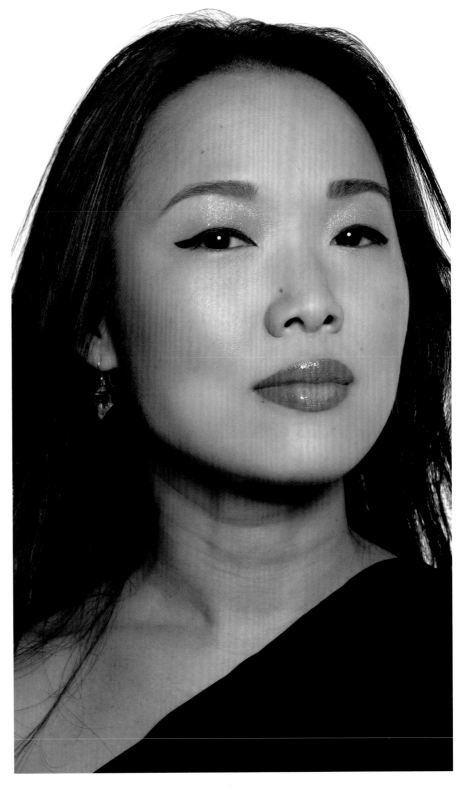

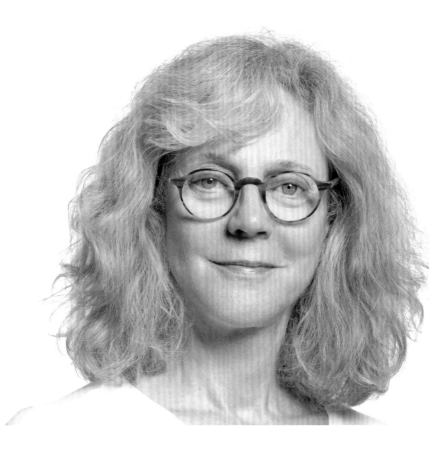

BLYTHE DANNER
ACTRESS

When Blythe came in for her photo shoot, she was incredibly open and trusting and had a *Let's do it!* attitude. She said, "I'm in your hands," and had so much fun with the process. Blythe was as comfortable with no makeup on as she was in her final outfit. When Blythe got on stage to have her picture taken, she lit up and began dancing. She has a natural grace and exuberance (plus some great moves). Everyone fell in love with Blythe.

—

Blythe has an iconic face and is blessed with beautiful piercing blue eyes and great skin. Pretty pink blush and lipstick immediately bring out Blythe's inner vibrancy. On her eyes, I used a light ivory shadow as a base and a soft taupe gray on the lid. Midnight navy shadow, applied with a damp eyeliner brush on the top lash line, makes her eyes stand out without being overpowering.

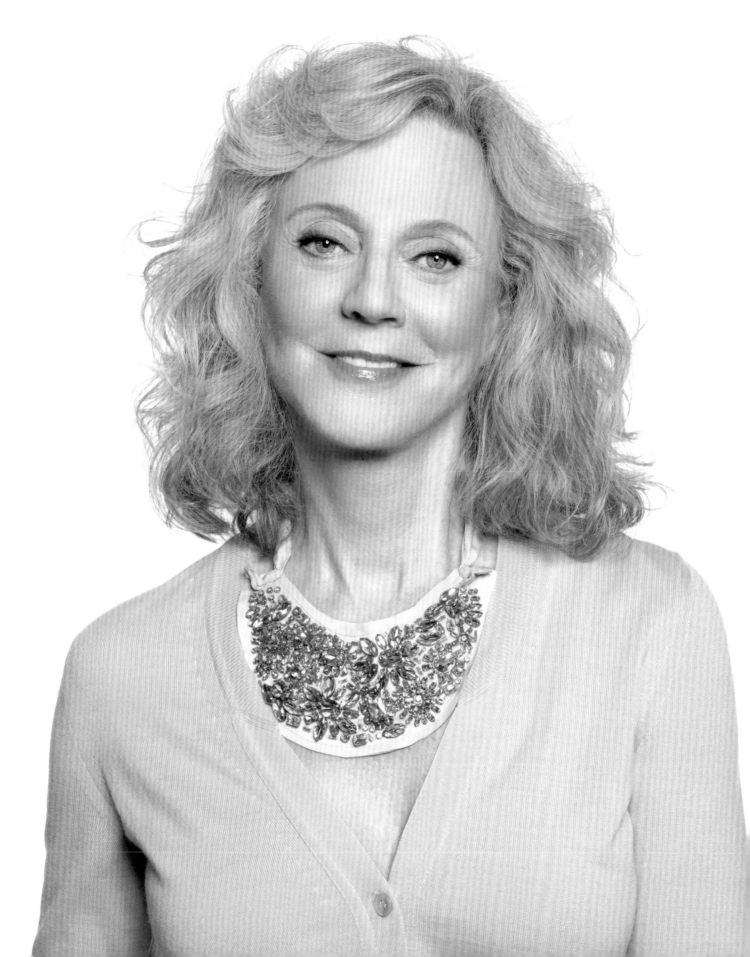

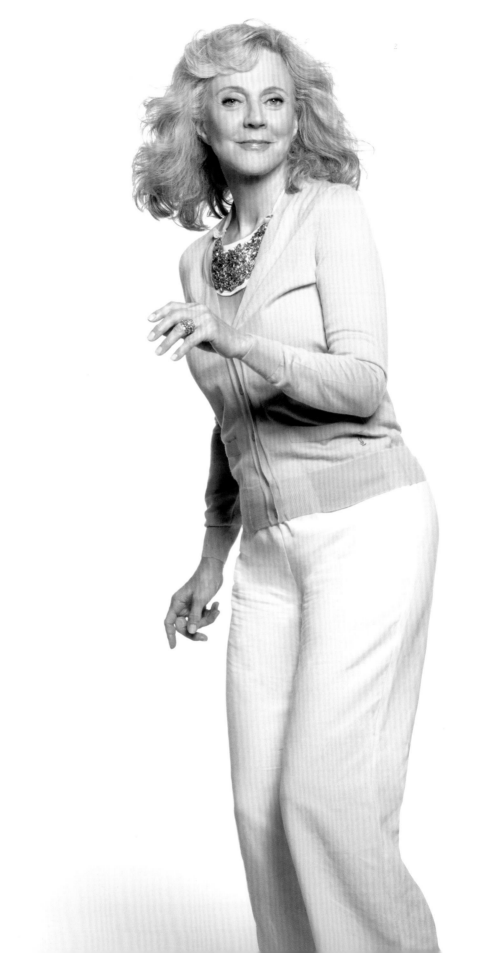

I've learned that to be negative about anything is such a waste.

—BLYTHE DANNER

I feel pretty when I'm getting made up. I love going from looking plain-Jane to looking gorgeous.

The best beauty advice I got was to stand up straight.

The best career advice is to persevere. As Chekhov said, "It's not the fame and the glory, it's the work."

My can't-live-without makeup is lipstick. My husband used to say women can't live without diamonds, but all I ever wanted was real estate and lipstick.

I feel powerful when I'm on stage.

My husband, Bruce, was the strongest, most extraordinary person that I ever met in my life. The wonderful thing about Bruce was that he gave so much to so many people. Now when we think of him, it is always in a restorative and very life-giving way. I still have people come up to me and say that he changed their life.

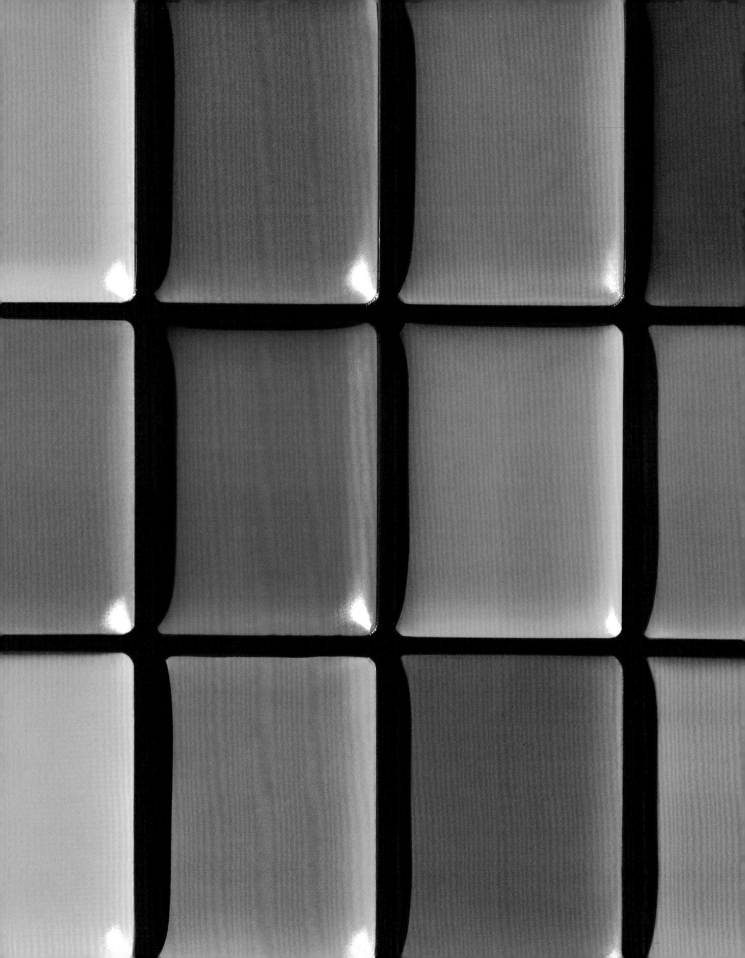

05

PRETTY AUTHENTIC

PRETTY AUTHENTIC

Women who are Pretty Authentic are honest, transparent, and full of integrity. They are who they are. Rose Cali, who is featured in this section, epitomizes all these qualities. Rose taught me that laughter is the best way to get through life. When I do too much or when things get messy, we laugh about it. She is a nurturer by nature and always giving, from cooking for her friends and family to her work as a community activist. Rose is not only a friend, but also a role model for me as a mother and philanthropist and how she lives her life on a daily basis.

Women who are Pretty Authentic often have the same friends, and sometimes the same style, for years. They tend to stick to what they love and only adopt trends that are right for them. The danger in this is that authentic women can sometimes find themselves in a style rut because they are too complacent and comfortable. So an update every two years or so is a good rule of thumb. I love to surround myself with women who are authentic (most of my closest friends fit into this category). Authentic women are amazing role models.

AUTHENTIC BEAUTY

Being authentic means playing up your best features to express who you are

———

DAY

SKIN

Depending on your skin type, choose a foundation that provides some coverage but is still sheer enough that you see your skin through it. If there is still any redness, apply cover-up stick on spots. If you have freckles, don't try to hide them with makeup, embrace them—they add so much character. Use a light undereye concealer if needed.

CHEEKS

Bronzer is an easy way to add color and warmth to the face. For a healthy glow, apply it where the sun naturally hits your skin—cheeks, forehead, nose, chin, and neck. If you have freckles, I love the combination of warm bronzer and apricot blush or the pretty juxtaposition of brown freckles with pink lips and cheeks.

EYES

There are many ways to make your eyes stand out—a sweep of shimmer, a bold liner, a combination of great colors. However, if you already have big, beautiful eyes, they don't need a lot of makeup to pop. White shadow is a subtle way to draw attention to your eyes. Paired with liner, a white matte powder for day and a white shimmer for night can be all you need to spotlight stunning eyes.

LIPS

There are tons of incredible shades to choose from to enhance your lips. An interesting way to highlight your lips is to play with texture within a range of natural shades that work with your coloring.

HAIR

Hair is one of those things that so many people start out fighting—trying to make thin hair thick, straight hair curly, brown hair blonde. But when you make peace with it and celebrate the hair you were born with, it starts to actually become one of your best assets. (Although a few high or low lights do help.)

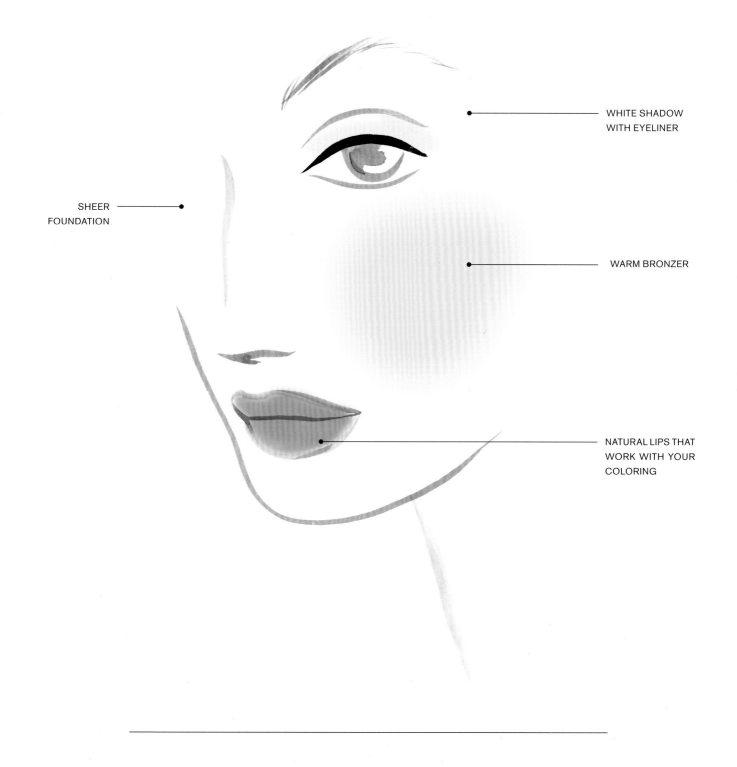

WHITE SHADOW
WITH EYELINER

SHEER
FOUNDATION

WARM BRONZER

NATURAL LIPS THAT
WORK WITH YOUR
COLORING

AUTHENTIC BEAUTY

Amp it up while still being you

——

EVENING

SKIN

For night, a little more coverage creates a polished look. However, it is so important to find the right texture; you want to look for a creamy but definitely natural finish.

CHEEKS

Layered on top of bronzer, a nectar or pink blush will brighten up the face.

EYES

Choosing soft, subtle shimmer for night, possibly in a cooler hue, paired with a liner and a few coats of mascara, highlights your eyes in a way that is pretty, not overpowering.

LIPS

For night, experiment with texture—a shimmery lipstick, a shiny colored gloss, or a sophisticated matte lip color. Even if it is the same color as your day lip, a different texture will change your look drastically.

HAIR

A great blowout with a bit of curl or soft waves will make a huge difference.

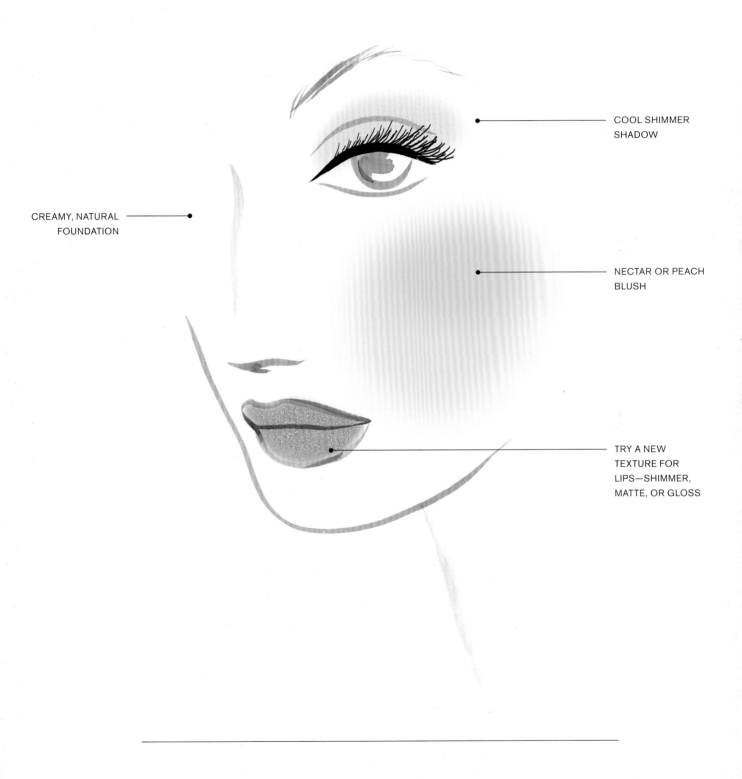

COOL SHIMMER
SHADOW

CREAMY, NATURAL
FOUNDATION

NECTAR OR PEACH
BLUSH

TRY A NEW
TEXTURE FOR
LIPS—SHIMMER,
MATTE, OR GLOSS

LEE WOODRUFF
WRITER, PUBLIC SPEAKER,
ADVOCATE FOR WOUNDED MILITARY HEROES

——

Not only is Lee the woman that everyone would love to have as a best friend—she's funny, bubbly, and happens to be a dancing dynamo—but she is also an incredible role model. After her husband, ABC News anchor Bob Woodruff, experienced a traumatic brain injury, they both used the difficult experience to inspire and help others. Lee and Bob coauthored their account of surviving the ordeal in the book *In an Instant*. They also founded the Bob Woodruff Foundation (REMIND.org) to help wounded servicemen and their families receive care and reintegrate into their communities.

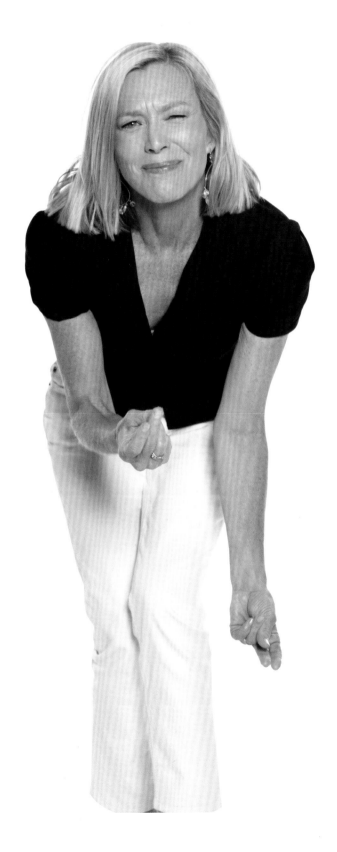

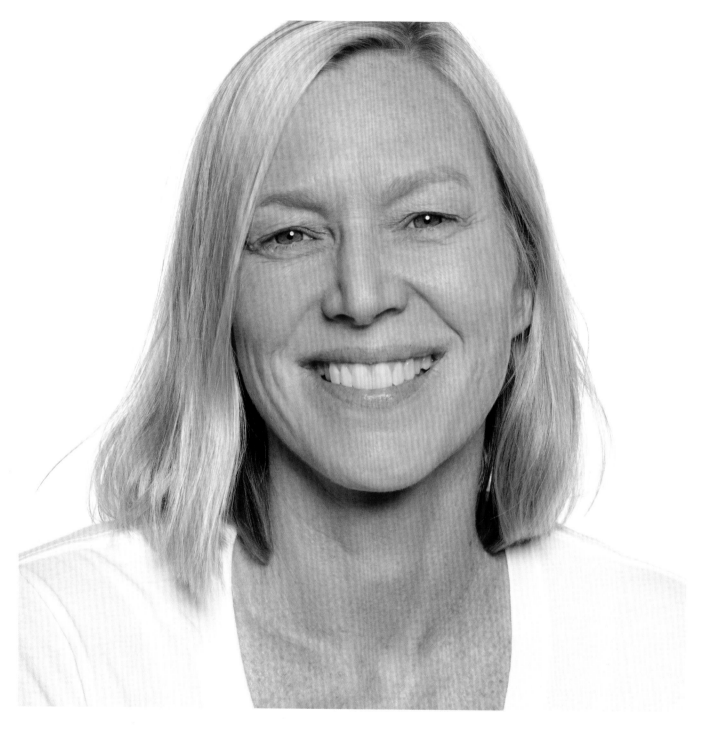

LEE WITHOUT MAKEUP

Barefaced, Lee looks like a very outdoorsy and fresh girl next door. Lee's great smile and sparkling eyes reflect her lively, vibrant energy.

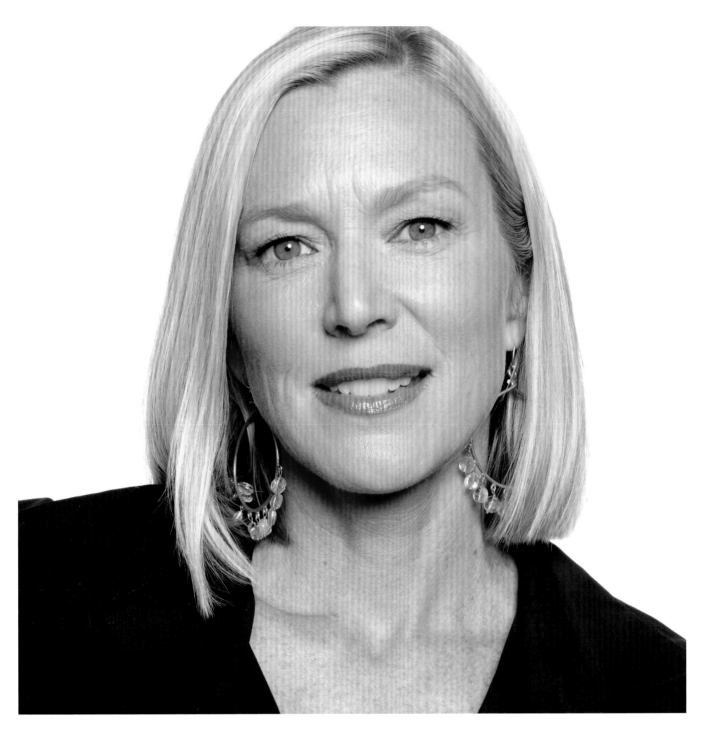

LEE WITH MAKEUP

Lee has an easy, natural beauty that we wanted to enhance but not overpower, so we relied on subtle colors. We started with a moisturizing foundation to even out her skin and still let her pretty freckles shine through. To bring out the wonderful shape of her eyes, we used a soft nude eye shadow and a caviar gel liner. A rosy cheek and lip color contrast beautifully with Lee's soft blonde hair. The result is a pretty, polished look that can work for day or night.

I feel powerful when I can do something good for somebody else.

—LEE WOODRUFF

My husband, Bob, was critically injured while covering the Iraq war. He really shouldn't be alive today. He was in a coma for thirty-six days in the hospital with a traumatic brain injury. I had to somehow stay positive and hopeful and show our four children that good things can come out of bad and that there's always hope even though I didn't feel it every day. I drew strength from so many things, from family and friends, from faith, and we got through it. He's recovered. He's back at work. We have an amazing life. We're lucky people.

I feel powerful when I can do something good for somebody else. When somebody calls me and their son has just been in a car accident, I can tell them that it will get better, that they will laugh again, that they will smile again. It makes me feel powerful to use what I know now and help somebody else who is just stepping onto the treadmill.

I am proud of being able to raise good, healthy, pretty cool kids and continue to do the work that I love. To write and do something creative and show your kids that you can love what you do, use your good in the world to help people, and use your creative juices to fulfill yourself is a wonderful feeling.

Nobody's perfect. We're doing the best we can and life is perfectly imperfect, so I just try to do what I can every day and not beat myself up.

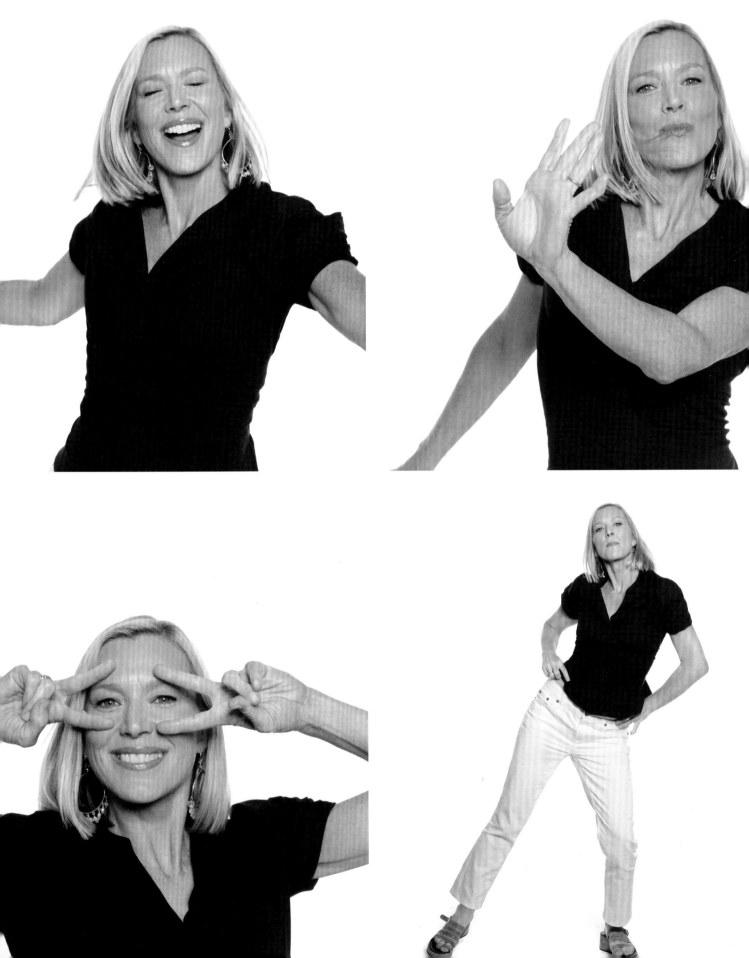

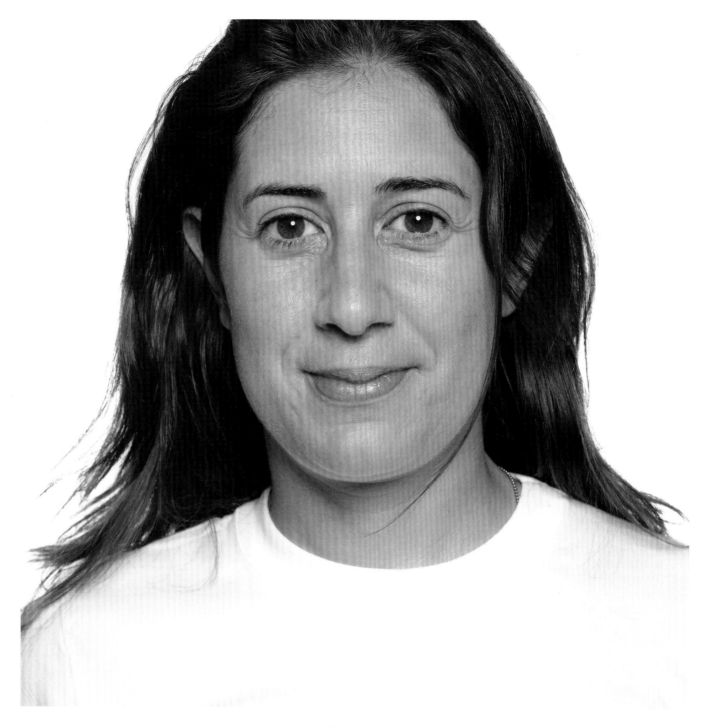

SUE TORRES CHEF

For me, power comes from physical strength. When I work out and am able to accomplish incredible things at the gym, I feel powerful. That energy carries on throughout the day.

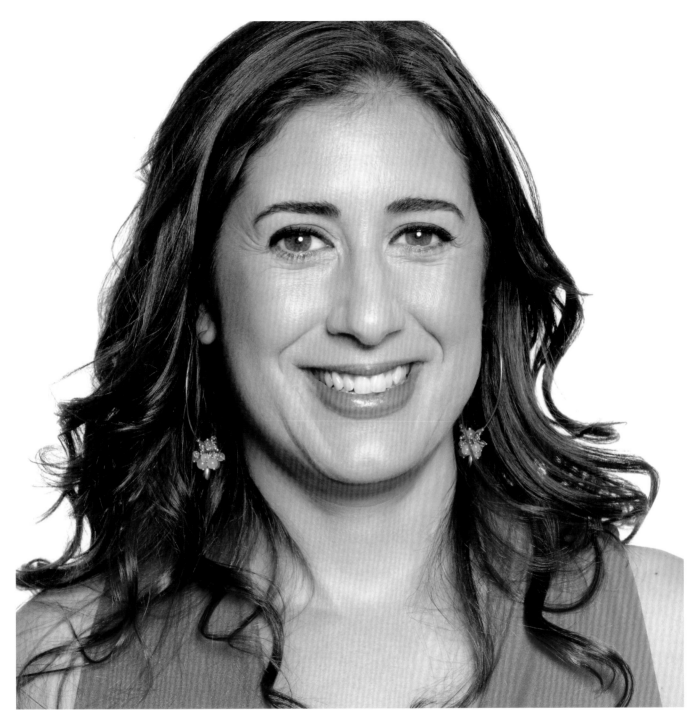

SUE'S MAKEUP

A chocolate-brown eyeliner is a good choice for accentuating dark brown eyes like Sue's. The shade complements her natural coloring beautifully, matching the depth of her brows and rich dark brown hair. Rosy lips complement her warm complexion.

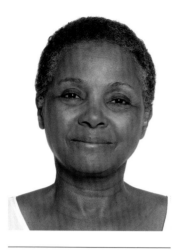

GRANVILETTE KESTENBAUM
MOTHER

I've always liked my smile. It's never the wrong size, never goes out of style, and always matches everything. The best part is that I can share my smile with others— there's always enough happiness to go around.

GRANVILETTE'S MAKEUP

What I love about Granvilette's makeover is that the colors work beautifully with her gorgeous skin tone. A cranberry pot rouge brings a fantastic brightness to her cheeks, while a medium brown lip color paired with a golden-pink shimmer gloss highlights her warm smile.

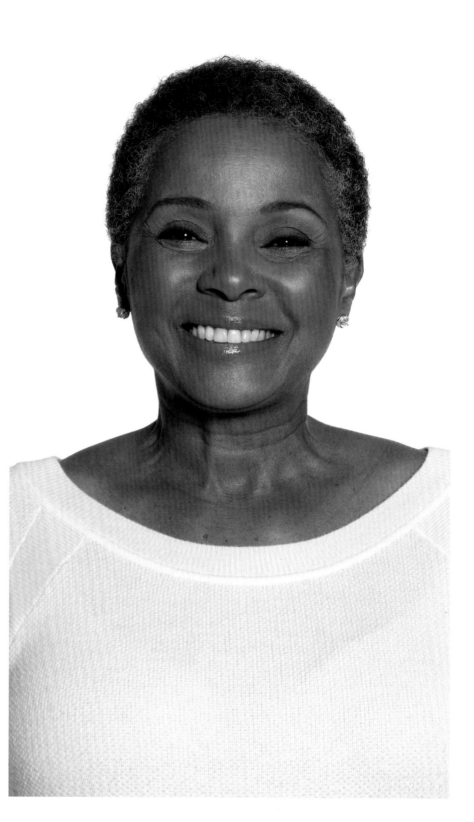

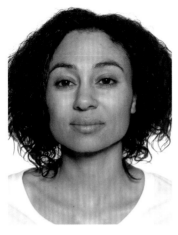

LAUREN KESTENBAUM
LAWYER

Every emotion I have is expressed through my face. So those who know me best can see when I'm having a good day, a bad day, or somewhere in between.

LAUREN'S MAKEUP

When you want your eyes to stand out more, line both top and bottom lashes; the trick is to make the top line stronger and the bottom line softer and have both lines meet at the outer corner. A strong line of black gel liner drawn across the full extent of Lauren's upper lash line and a softer black shadow on the bottom bring drama to her stunning eyes. Keeping lips and cheeks in soft rosy-pink tones lets Lauren's eyes steal the spotlight. Lauren's gorgeous curly hair frames her face beautifully.

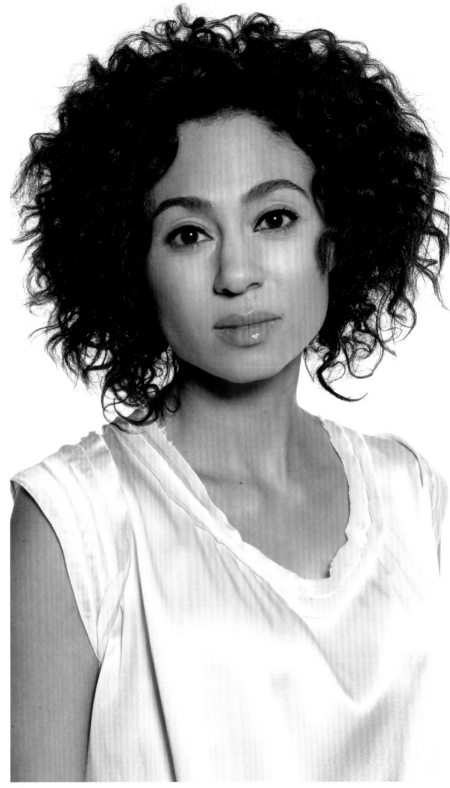

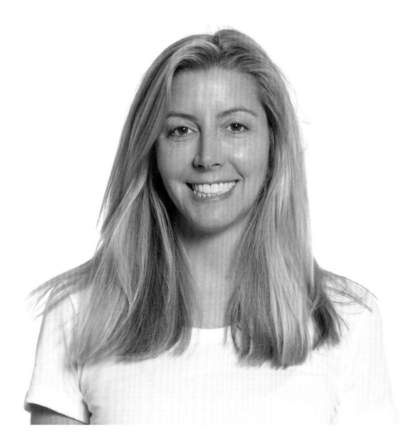

SARA BLAKELY
ENTREPRENEUR

Sara has classic, fresh-faced looks and a friendly, outgoing personality. I love that she also happens to be a total powerhouse. Her product, Spanx, has become a common noun in America—the same way people call all tissues Kleenex, people now refer to all shape-wear as Spanx. The magic of her product is that it is a great self-esteem enhancer and confidence builder for millions of women.

—

With her big smile, bubbly and open personality, and beautiful blonde hair, Sara stands out naturally. To let Sara be the one to shine and not her makeup, I went with softer colors than she normally wears. I swept a shimmery ivory over lids with a subtle hint of gray shimmer in the crease. I lined her eyes with a grayish-black gel eyeliner. The pinky nude tones on Sara's lips and cheeks illuminate her warm smile.

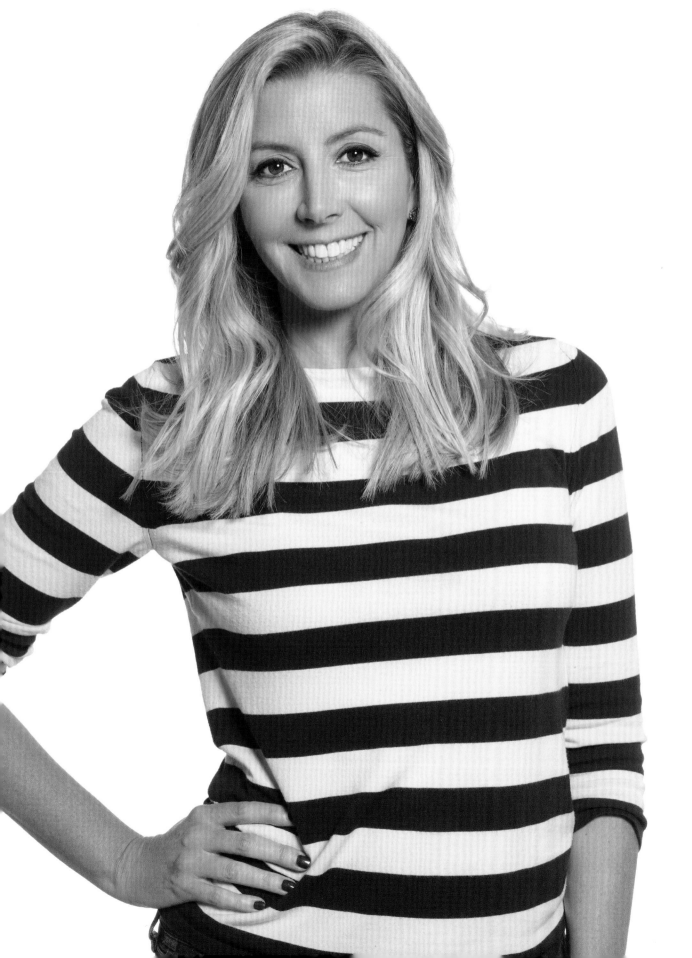

I'm proud that I've been able to become successful while being kind to people.

—SARA BLAKELY

My father used to encourage us to fail when we were younger. We would sit at the dinner table and he would ask us what we had failed at that week, and if we didn't have anything, he would be disappointed. It was one of the biggest gifts in my life because it taught my brother and me not to be afraid of failing. It meant we were constantly pushing ourselves out of the box and trying new things. For me the definition of failure is not trying, not the outcome. The only time I feel like I'm failing is if I don't do something because I am afraid.

I'm a new mom, and juggling and navigating motherhood and my career and the balance of it all—it's a tough thing to figure out. I'm still a work in progress.

I'm proud that I've been able to become successful while being kind to people. I feel like I did it in a way that I can look in the mirror now and feel really good about how I got to where I am.

Being able to follow my own path and answer only to myself is a very powerful feeling.

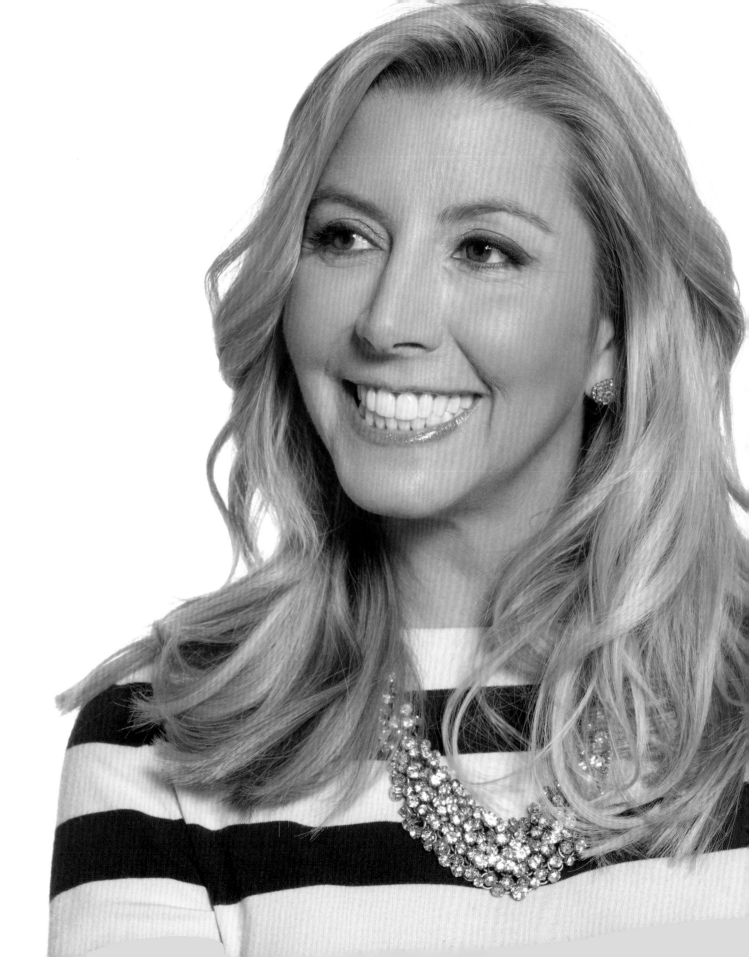

BE WHO YOU ARE

In the nineties, I was working at a fashion show with several top supermodels. I was about fifteen years older than many of them and pregnant with my first son. I remember looking up at all these young, tall, perfect women, who happened to be wearing bikinis, and feeling very short and very big. At the same time, there was also a voice in my head saying, *Don't go there, Bobbi. This is not a competition that you can win. Let it go.* It was my "aha" moment. I realized that, I needed to accept who I was—thirty years old, five feet tall, and beautifully pregnant. I was lucky to be doing a job I loved, lucky to be me— exactly as I was.

The fashion and beauty industry is filled with the most stunning women in the world. It would be very easy to get caught up in an unrealistic view of reality, but if I start to feel insecure, I just remind myself who I am—an involved mom of three boys, a devoted wife, an artist who is also the head of a giant company, a fun friend, and (just like everyone) imperfect. I strive to be honest and nice, always. I am the same whether I am hanging out with my boys at home, meeting with a top editor, or getting a celebrity ready for the red carpet. I wear worn-in jeans most days. Some mornings, I come to work with wet hair pulled back into a ponytail. And forget stilettos; I save those for the red carpet or high-profile events after dark. I am most comfortable in clogs or Converse sneakers. That's who I am and I couldn't be happier about it.

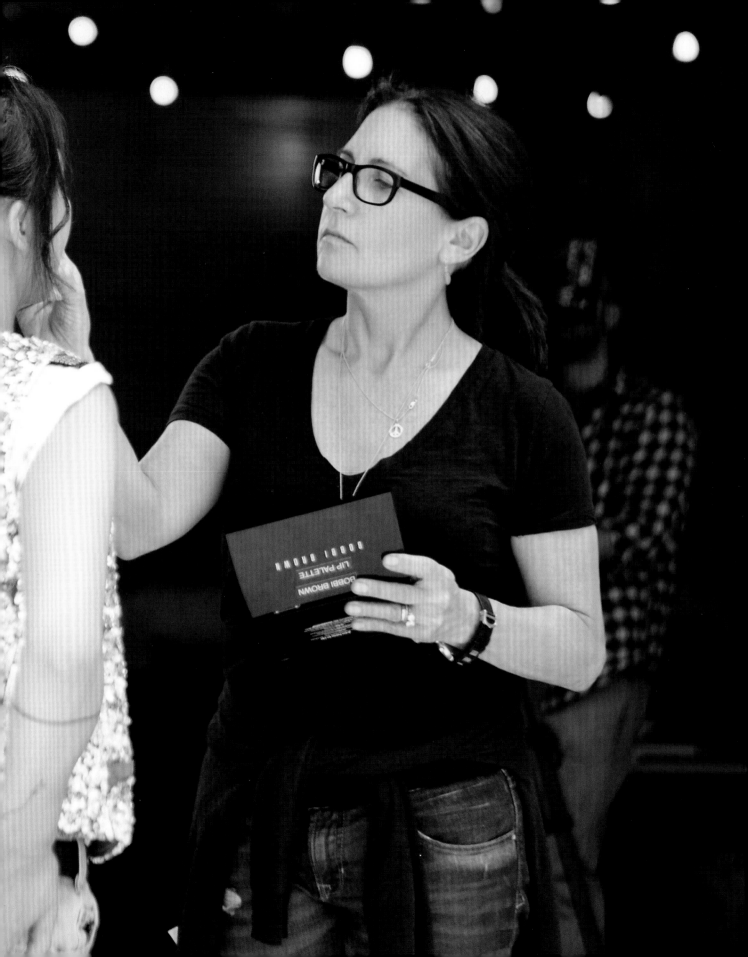

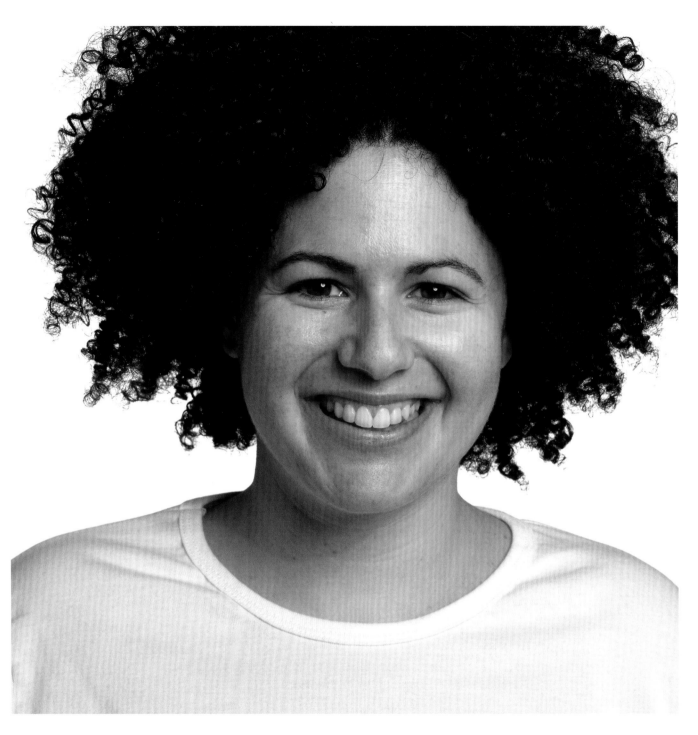

LAUREN RIFKIN
DIRECTOR OF ONLINE MARKETING AND E-COMMERCE
My husband told me that I have flowers in my eyes. It's the best compliment I've ever received.

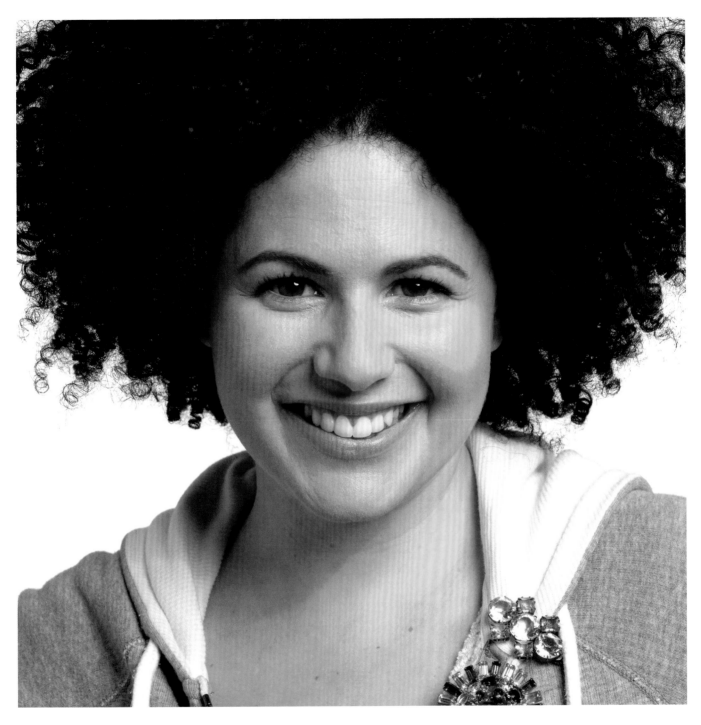

LAUREN'S MAKEUP

Lauren lets her gorgeous curly hair steal the spotlight, but she is a minimalist when it comes to makeup. We kept her makeup light, just applying a stick foundation to eliminate any touches of redness, setting it with a dusting of yellow-based powder. Adding bronzer and a pop of a peony-colored blush created a healthy glow. For her eyes, we swept creamy pinkish-white all over her lids along with a black gel liner and a few coats of black mascara. Simple and beautiful.

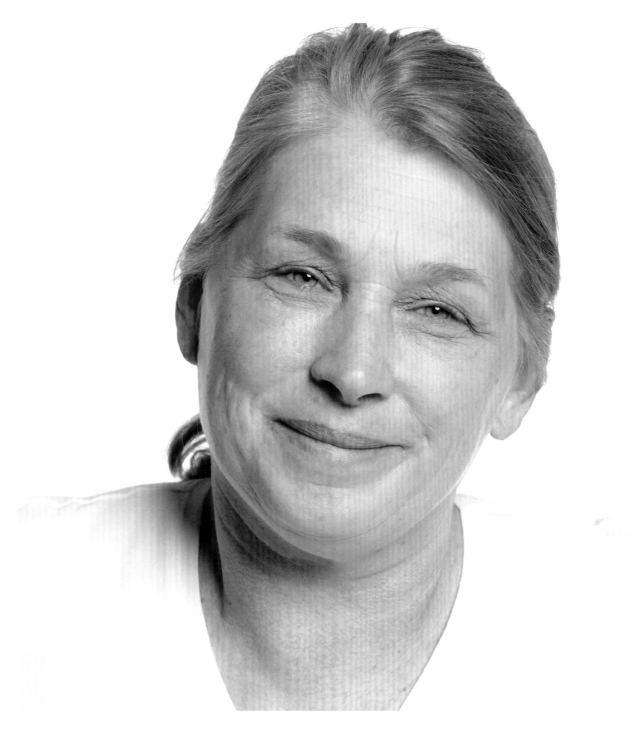

BETH BALDWIN BREAST CANCER CRUSADER

*I think the determination that all my siblings and I have is that you can do anything you want
to do; you just have to make that choice to do it. I've taught my children the same thing.*

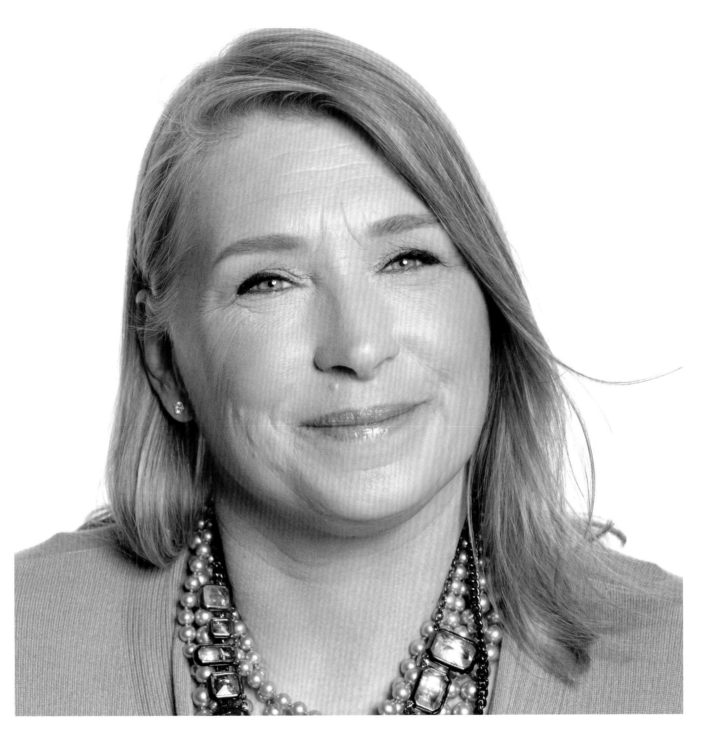

BETH'S MAKEUP

For Beth, I concentrated on bringing out her inner sparkle. A glossy pink lip, rose pot rouge on cheeks, and champagne shimmer eye shadow adds luminosity that suits Beth perfectly.

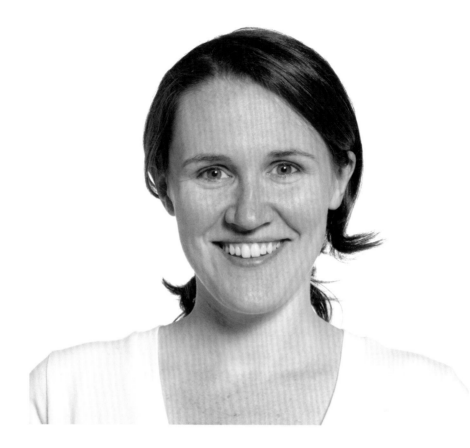

LIZ MURRAY
AUTHOR, MOTIVATIONAL SPEAKER

When I read Liz Murray's book *Breaking Night*, I couldn't put it down. I was stunned and moved by her story of growing up with drug-addicted parents, surviving homelessness, and making it to Harvard. At the photo shoot for the book, Liz arrived with her adorable husband and best friend. She was seven months pregnant with her first child and glowing. Despite the tough experiences Liz was handed in life, she rose above it all and has made an incredible life for herself empowering other women. She is such an inspiration.

—

When you have beautiful, deep-set eyes like Liz, the trick is to stick with lighter eye shadows to bring them out. An ivory shadow all over her lid opens her eyes while a softer black gel liner creates definition. On both the top and bottom lash line, I smudged espresso-brown liner for a softer effect that not only illuminates her expressive, soulful eyes, but highlights her warm personality without overpowering her natural beauty.

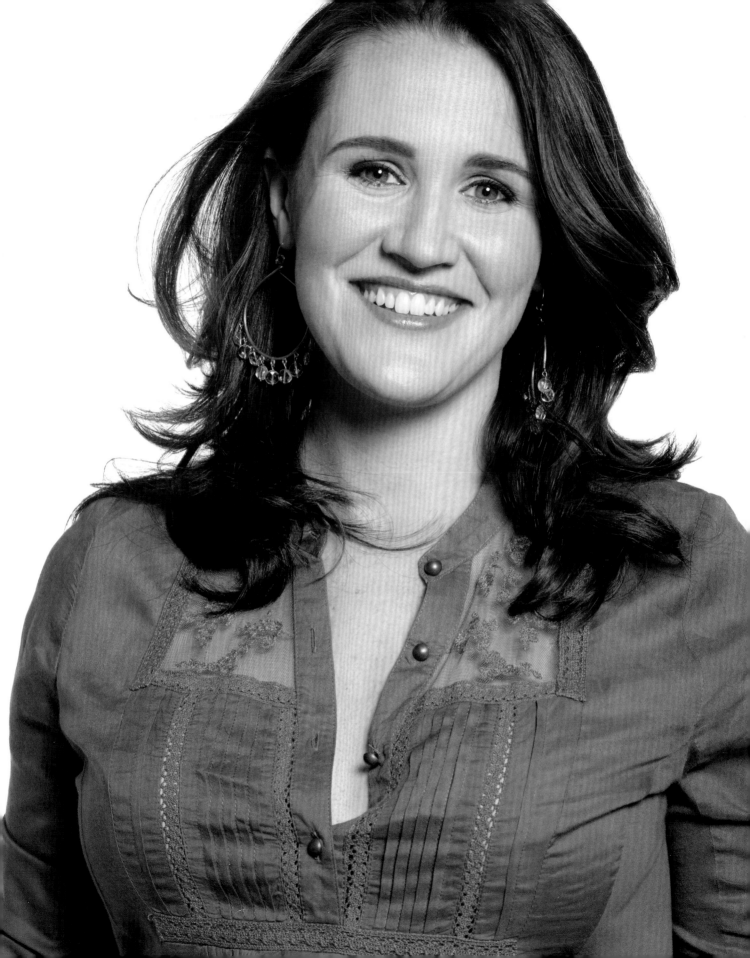

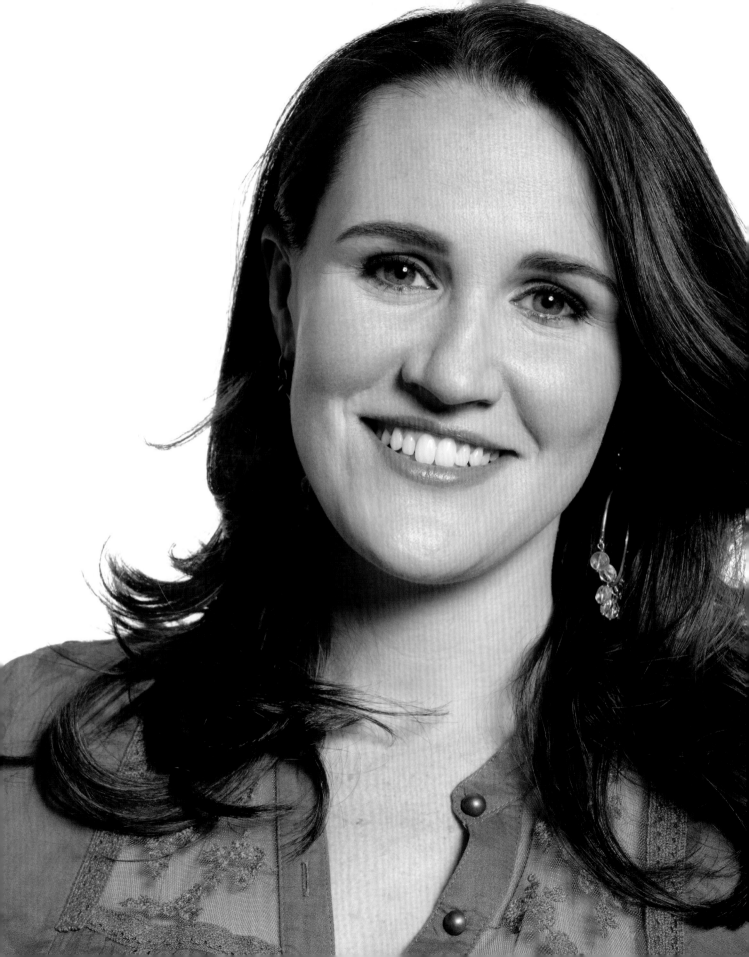

You can change your life. In fact, you can transform your life.

—LIZ MURRAY

I feel powerful when I give myself permission to be authentic. The times in my life when I would look around the room and try to decide what I should say or what I should be—based on what I thought others might want of me—I wasn't in my power. I'm most fierce when I just call on what's inside of me and I'm simply myself.

I was homeless for a while. I was living on the streets and I remember just waiting for things to happen. I would wait for a sign for something to send me back to school. I would wait to change my life. Losing my mom was a profoundly painful experience, but it was also eye-opening. When I lost her I got in touch with mortality. I just realized, *What am I waiting for? My life is happening right now.* I learned to just go for things. Now I recognize that when I tell myself I'll do it later, that's actually just a lie. I don't wait anymore. Now when there's something that's meaningful to me, I don't take for granted that I could do it tomorrow, I just go for it.

I'm expecting my first child. It is sort of emotional because when I think about the next ten years, I want to fill a dinner table. I want to have noise and clatter in my house. I want to look up and see the people that I love and know that they're close to me and that we can reach each other. That would be a beautiful life.

If you go through things where you feel like you're in a dark place, you are not alone. That really is just a human experience and life doesn't have to be that way. You can change your life. In fact, you can transform your life. If I could go back to myself when I was homeless at fifteen, I would just tell myself, *This is something you're going through. You're not alone. There is a way out. There's going to be a life beyond this and it is going to be awesome.*

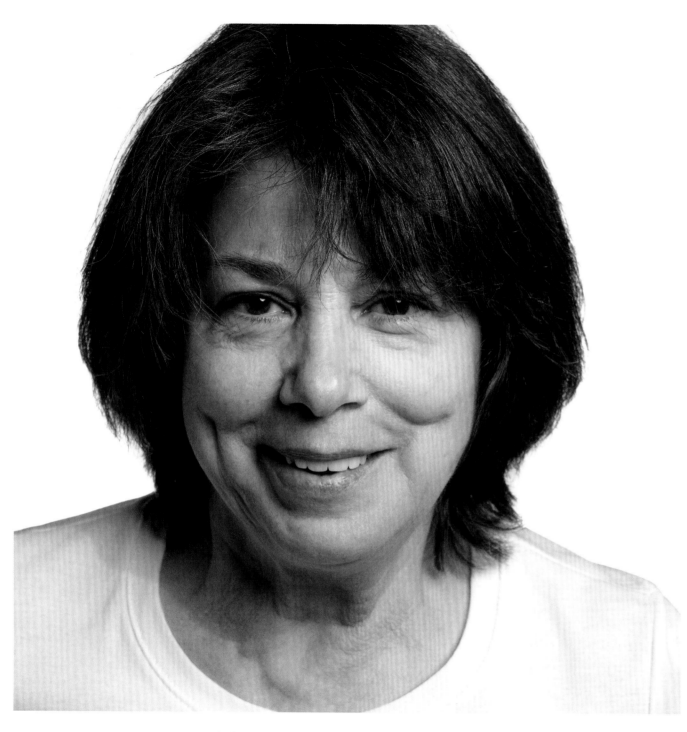

ROSE CALI COMMUNITY ACTIVIST

The best beauty advice I've ever gotten was from Bobbi: Be who you are.

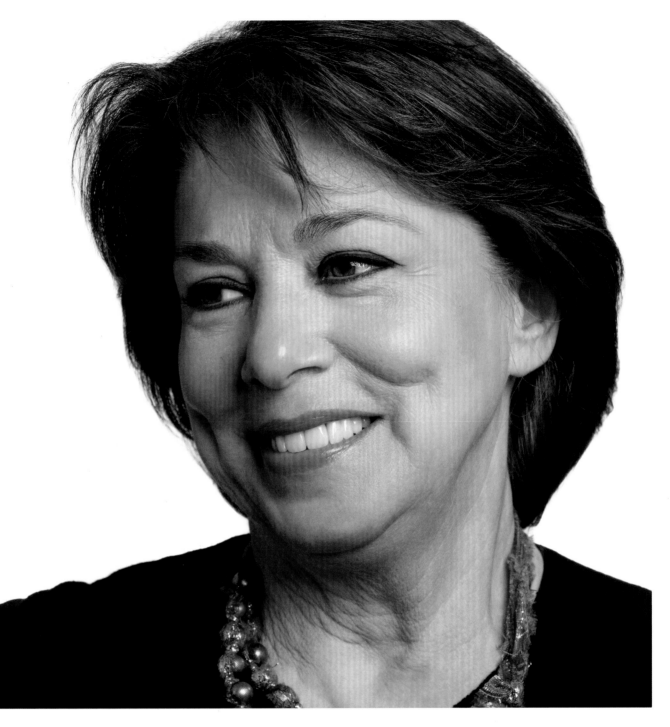

ROSE'S MAKEUP

Rose is my son's godmother, my life role model, and one of the warmest people I know. To highlight her great smile and wonderful dimples, I relied on bronzer and a pop of pale pink blush. Dimples are a feature I like to celebrate—they add so much personality. The Italian Rose lipstick that she is wearing is named after her.

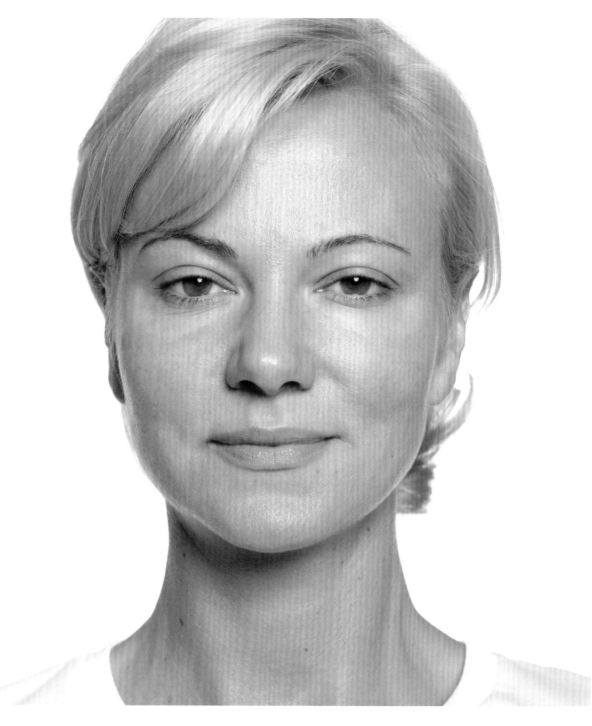

SARMA MELNGAILIS RAW FOOD GURU

A process women go through as they age is that they start to feel more comfortable in their own skin. It would be great to find a way to make that happen earlier. I wish when I was younger I had a better appreciation of myself and didn't worry so much about what people thought.

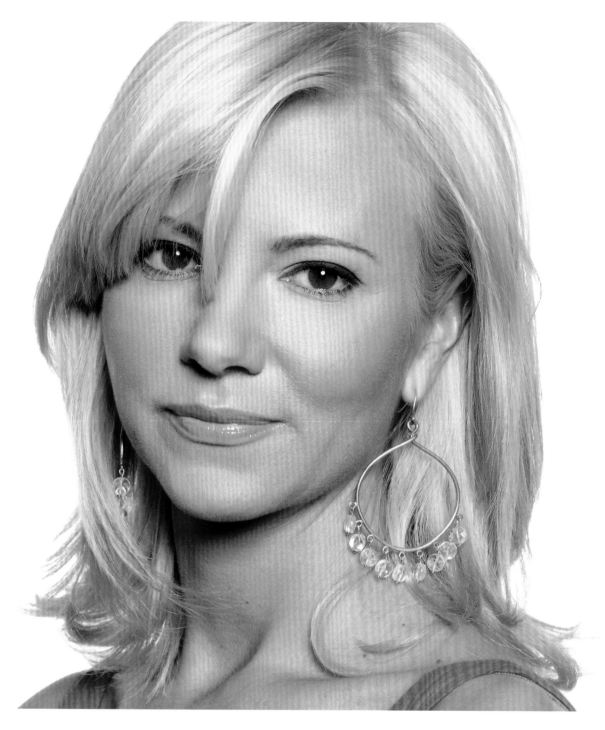

SARMA'S MAKEUP

When you have striking blonde hair, brown eyes, and fair skin like Sarma, you need to add color to your face to avoid looking washed out. A warm-toned foundation and bronzer, followed by a pink blush on the apples of the cheeks, give Sarma a vibrant glow and highlight her striking features. A gray shadow brings depth to her brows, while a soft black gel liner layered with a navy shadow liner on the top lash line, along with a light application of navy shadow on the lower lash line, is a pretty way to bring out her eyes.

SANDRA BERNHARD
ACTRESS, COMEDIAN

—

I originally met Sandra in Chicago at a fundraiser. She is undeniably hilarious with a sharp wit, which is to be expected, but Sandra's also warm, caring, down-to-earth, and totally nice. I love her "I am who I am" attitude. She possesses a strength and confidence that is so refreshing.

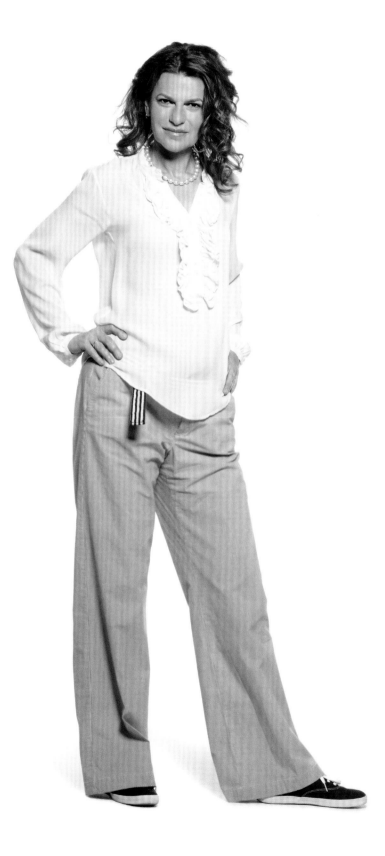

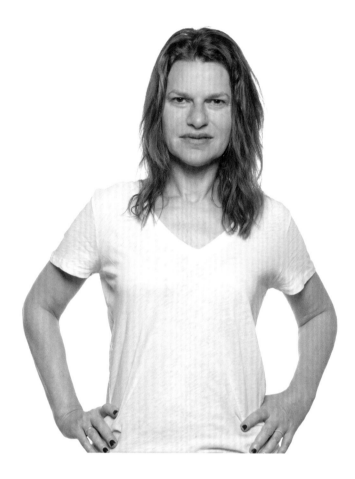

SANDRA WITHOUT MAKEUP

Sandra has a natural warmth and spark in her eyes and a beautiful, milky complexion.

SANDRA WITH MAKEUP

When you have a fair complexion like Sandra, a yellow-toned foundation can actually bring a bit of warmth to the skin. I love the juxtaposition of soft, romantic pale pink blush and lips with Sandra's beautiful, strong features and bold personality.

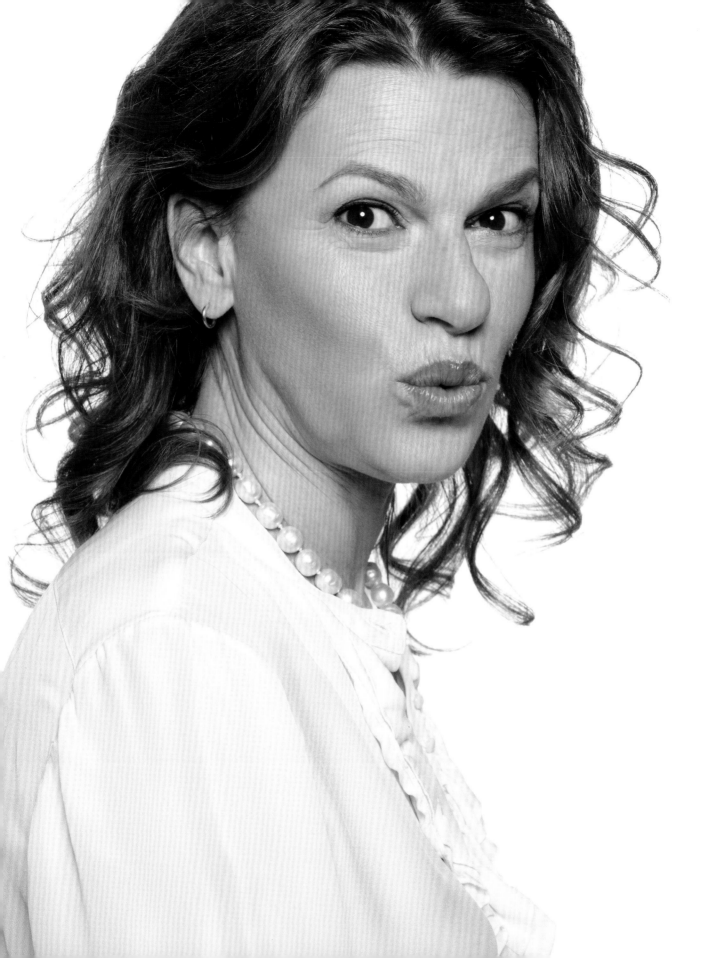

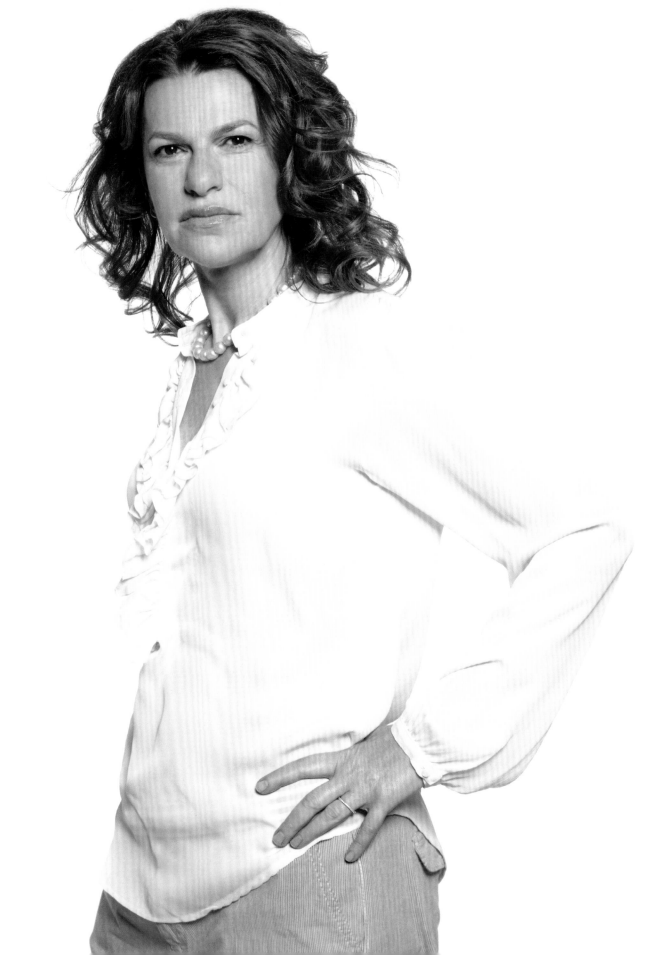

Power is having a clear point of view about what's important in your life.

—SANDRA BERNHARD

Day to day I think the greatest happiness is having a family. Having a daughter, my partner, my dog—just getting up in the morning and having these really special elements around me is wonderful and emotional.

The best beauty advice I ever received was don't overdo it. Don't take it too over the top.

My greatest indulgence is getting up in the middle of the night and eating things that I shouldn't eat.

Power is when you really tap into who you are and have complete and total confidence in yourself. Power is having a clear point of view about what's important in your life and your take on the world. Being a part of the world. Being compassionate. Being supportive of people's rights and freedoms. Being somebody who is willing to speak out when things are not right. I think that is the power we all possess, and as women, I think we have a bigger responsibility to help other people.

06

PRETTY BOLD

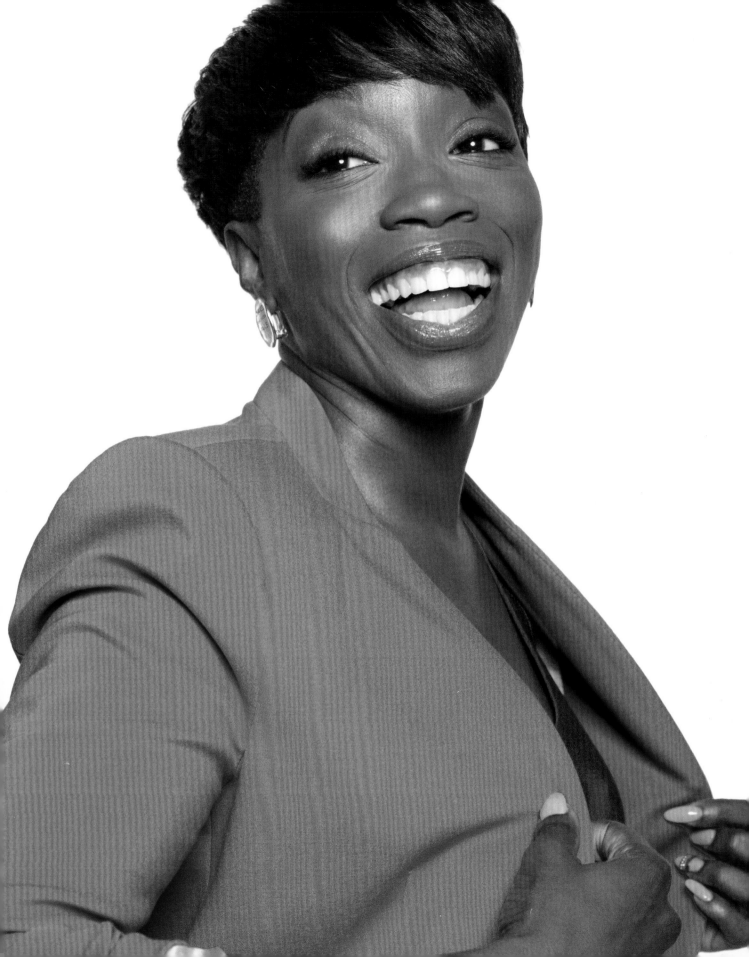

PRETTY BOLD

I admire women who are Pretty Bold. They pull things off that would make the rest of us look totally absurd. Madonna does this effortlessly. She's gone from the nineties pop icon who inspired many of us to punk out to a glamorous Hollywood starlet to an English lady of the manor—Madonna becomes whoever she wants to be. Lady Gaga and Nicki Minaj have followed in Madonna's footsteps. While I personally think that they both might look a bit more beautiful with a simpler style, these pop superstars are most happy to be who they are in that moment, and that is the point.

Boldness should not be confused with bad taste. Some women think wearing low-cut dresses or extremely short minis is being bold. But the trick is to be age-appropriate and, of course, comfortable. My own boldness comes out in different ways—from the Converse sneakers I wore to the White House to the Louboutin hot pink stilettos that I save for a pink party I attend every year, or wearing no makeup to an event (usually after a long Fashion Week), I sometimes go with my gut instead of what I'm expected to do. I love Pretty Bold women because, to quote Clark Gable, frankly my dear, they just don't give a damn.

BOLD MAKEUP

How to experiment with your look

———

DAY

SKIN

Women who are bold go from using no foundation some days to full coverage, depending on how they feel at the moment. As long as the foundation is the right tint and color for the skin, with yellow undertones, you can use any foundation you like.

CHEEKS

A bright pop of color on the cheeks paired with nude lips is eye-catching. For an instant glow, rub a clear balm on top of blush. Shimmer over blush brings a playful touch of sparkle to your cheekbones.

EYES

If you want to be a little rock 'n' roll with your eye makeup for day, it's okay to get creative and have fun. Line eyes with an unexpected shade like plum or violet, and smudge.

LIPS

There is something very cool about the contrast of a fresh face and a hot pink or neon orange lip. I also love the drama of beige lips paired with a smoky metallic eye.

HAIR

Because your beauty is so based on your personality and spirit, why not be adventurous when it comes to hair? Try a bold hair color or androgynous cut—go ahead, it grows out!

P.S.

Nails are a great (and noncommittal) place to be bold. Neon, white, chocolate, and navy are fun colors to play with. Promise me—just keep them short!

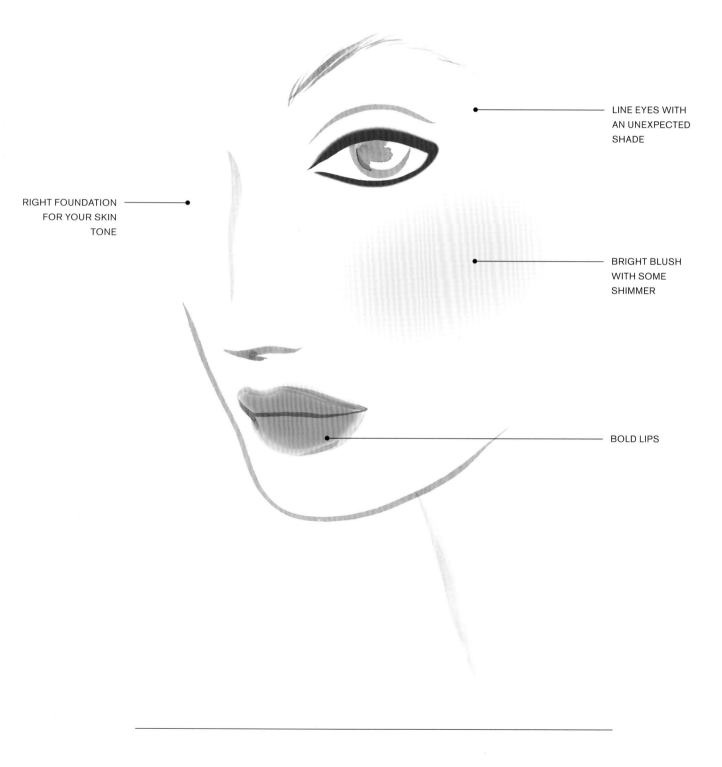

LINE EYES WITH
AN UNEXPECTED
SHADE

RIGHT FOUNDATION
FOR YOUR SKIN
TONE

BRIGHT BLUSH
WITH SOME
SHIMMER

BOLD LIPS

BOLD MAKEUP

Get creative and have fun

EVENING

SKIN

For bold women it's all about having fun and going with how you feel at the moment. Have a range of foundation types on hand to experiment with—from sheer to dewy to matte to full coverage.

CHEEKS

Cheeks should stay pretty much the same at night as for day; you could maybe add a bit more to adjust for lighting. Sometimes a punch of bright blended blush can be gorgeous with a pale lip and eye.

EYES

A dramatic smoky eye in unusual colors makes a sexy statement at night. Keep lips and cheeks neutral so that your eyes really stand out.

LIPS

Creating eye-catching lips means playing with color, anything from acid orange to violet to pale champagne. Just make sure the rest of the face is balanced. If your lips are the exclamation point for your look, keep your eyes a bit softer and vice versa.

HAIR

Do the unexpected, which can mean playing it down as much as playing it up. Soft, pretty hair contrasted with striking makeup is very contemporary and cool. Try slicked back and sleek, subtle and soft, or amp up your curls. Have fun!

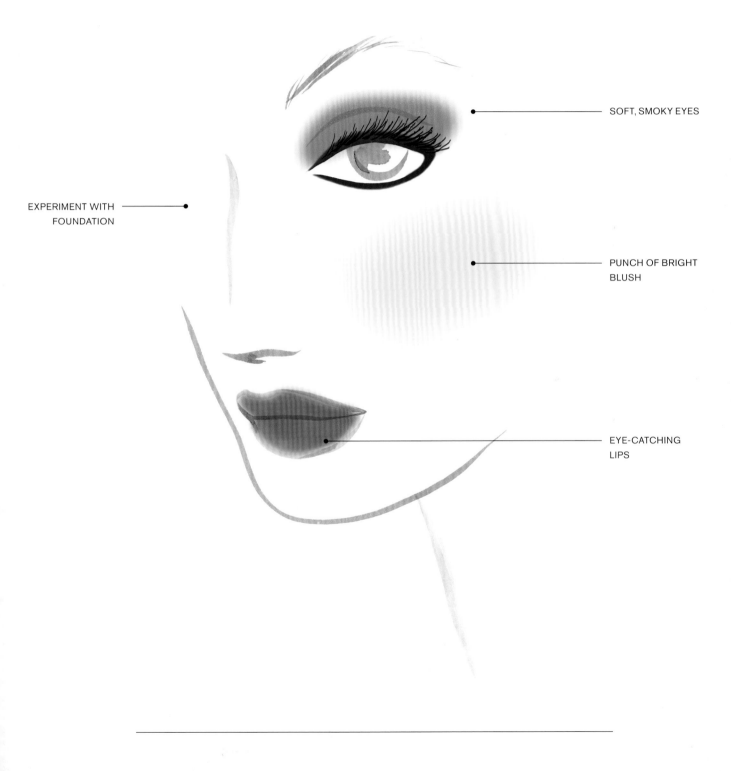

SOFT, SMOKY EYES

EXPERIMENT WITH
FOUNDATION

PUNCH OF BRIGHT
BLUSH

EYE-CATCHING
LIPS

ESTELLE
RECORDING ARTIST

———

When Estelle enters a room, she does it quietly. She's petite and sweet and doesn't demand attention, but it's impossible not to notice her. Estelle has stunning eyes, striking features, and a fierce short haircut that turns heads. She also gives off this really great energy. Estelle is at a very happy point in her life, and it shows. She has won a Grammy, she's working on new music, and she's made some changes with diet and exercise that have her glowing. Estelle is very alive and effortlessly cool. She's one of those people you want around all the time.

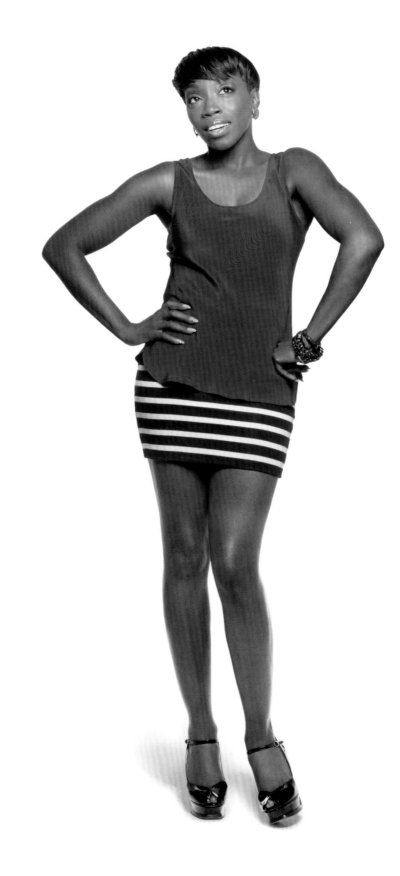

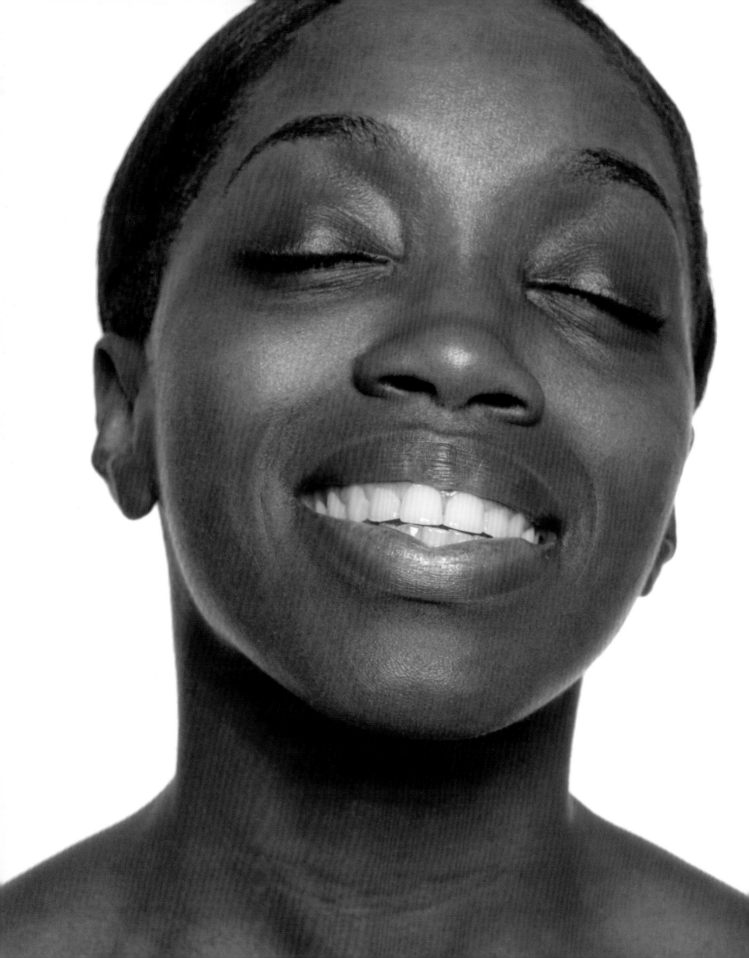

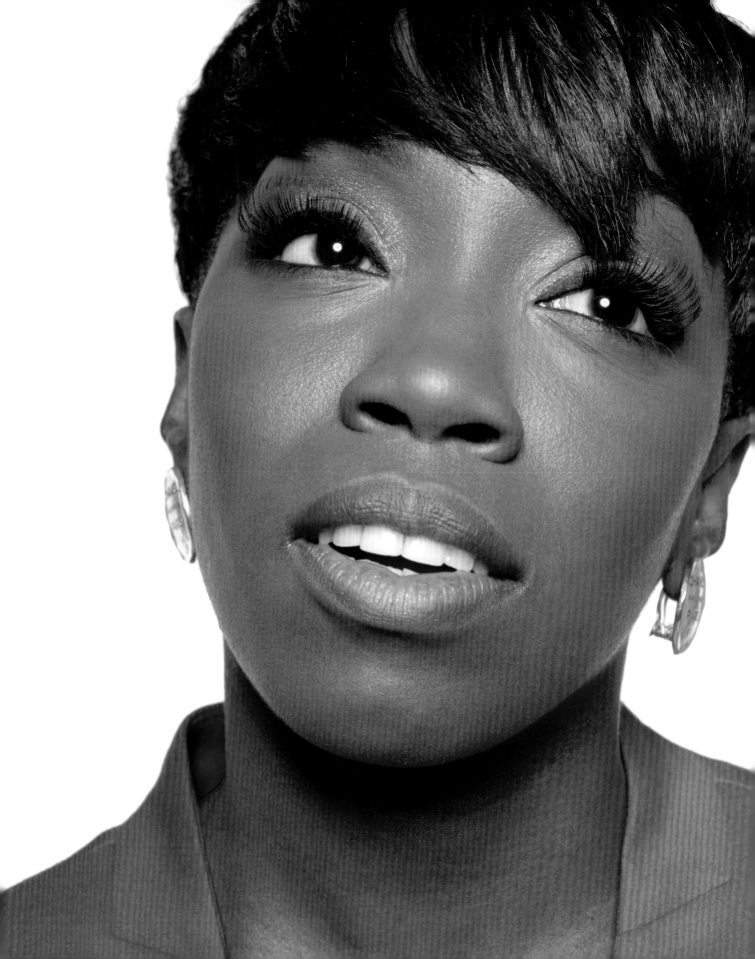

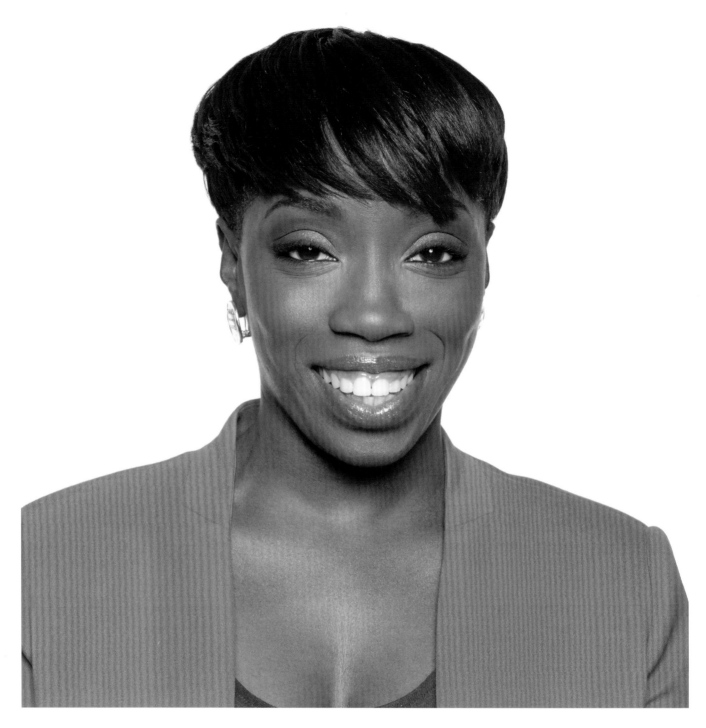

ESTELLE'S MAKEUP

I played up Estelle's amazing almond-shaped eyes with a plum shimmer shadow on the lids and a gener-
ous application of black gel liner on the top lash line. A thinner line of matte plum shadow on the bottom
lash line frames her eyes and works with her cool hair color. To enhance Estelle's show-stopping lashes,
I layered several coats of black lengthening mascara. With bold eyes I like to keep lips more subtle; for
Estelle, a beige lip gloss adds a subtle sparkle that complements her look.

My motto is "If you want it, go and get it."

—ESTELLE

When you've been told that you can't do something and all of a sudden it happens, it makes you feel like you've conquered the world.

I started as a rapper, so it was a challenge to become comfortable with my singing voice. I overcame that by taking singing from a place of my soul, versus trying to be technically correct or trying to be the best singer on the planet. I just decided to sing from my heart.

For about twenty years I didn't listen to the advice to drink water, but five years ago I started, and it really works. Water does everything. It helps with weight loss. It keeps your skin bright. It helps with energy levels. It really does a lot.

I have so many dreams for myself. I want to be married. I want to have some kids. I want to be an actress. I also want to do more behind-the-scenes stuff like producing. Those are my main goals, but I also want to do my photography on a professional level. I like catching people in the moment; I'm obsessed with those seventies pictures of people in the clubs. When I'm with my friends I have them keep talking and living while I take pictures because that's when you see real joy. I want to remember those moments. I'll definitely have an exhibit someday.

COMFORTABLE AND CONFIDENT

Now that I'm in my fifties, I have a confidence that has come with time and experience. The fifties have become the "I'm over it" decade. Relationships that were once either forced or superficial are let go of—there just isn't time. Plans not going the way you thought? Change them! Your body's not fitting into that once-sexy skintight dress? Go out and get one that's a bit looser, and at the same time, up your mileage on the treadmill. Be comfortable and be active, and I promise that you'll be confident.

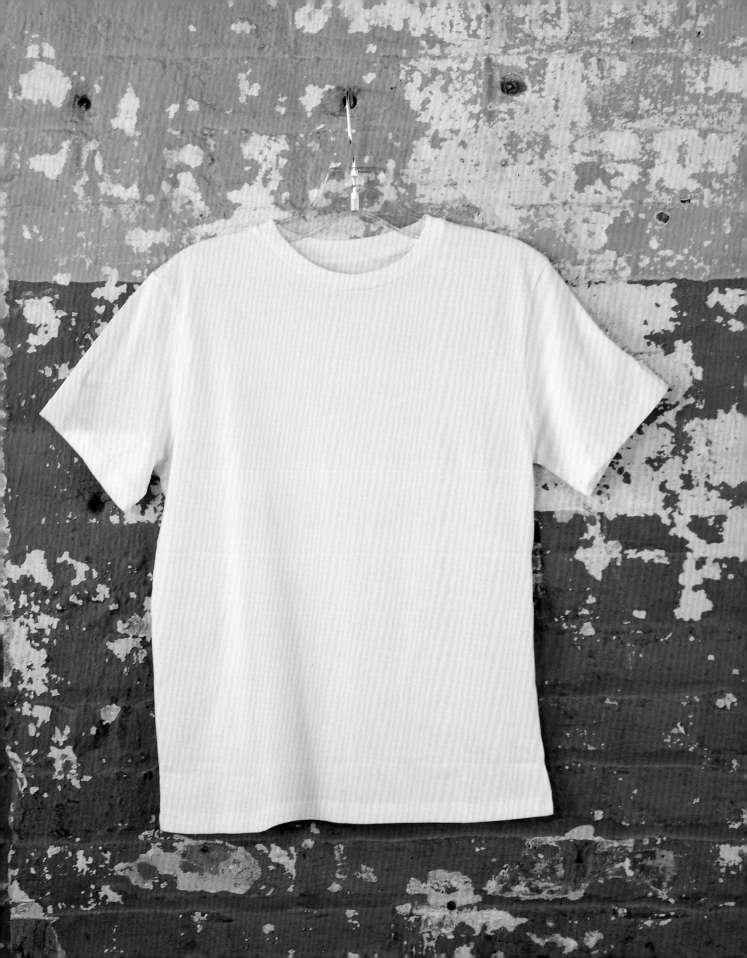

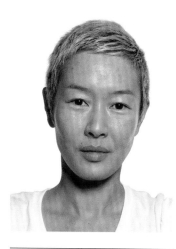

JENNY SHIMIZU
MODEL BOOKER, MODEL, MECHANIC

I like my differences; they are my strengths. My androgyny, my comfortableness in my own skin—these things I now honor.

JENNY'S MAKEUP— DAY

With her bleached blonde hair, dark eyes, and striking looks, Jenny doesn't need a lot of makeup to stand out. A light bronzing powder on cheeks, forehead, nose, chin, and neck paired with a pale pink blush gives Jenny a pretty subtle flush. Jenny's beautiful baby-doll pout makes a statement on its own, so we skipped color and opted for a sheer lip balm. For eyes, a sweep of sheer ivory metallic shimmer adds an iridescent glow. A black gel liner applied to her upper lash line and winged out at the edges adds a cool elongating effect that works with Jenny's cool style.

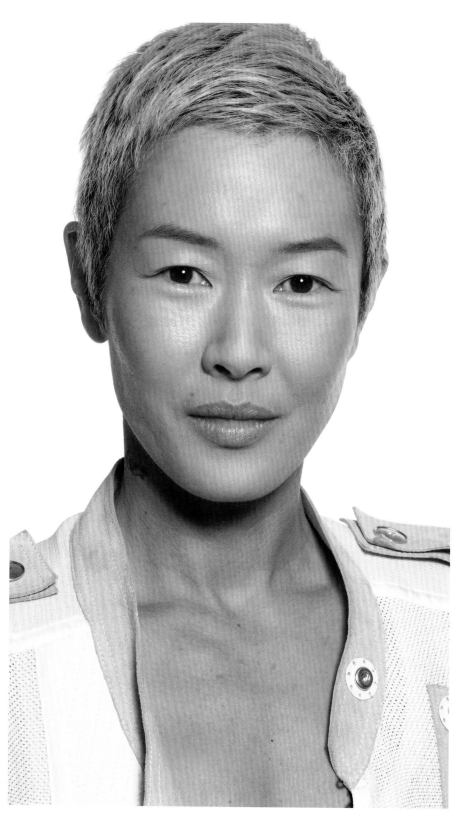

JENNY'S MAKEUP—
NIGHT

For a dramatic evening look, we focused on amping up Jenny's eyes. We swept a silver cream shadow over Jenny's entire lid and then blended a dark gray shadow from the lash line to the crease, layering the color until we got the perfect smoky look. On top of the black gel liner we smudged a char-coal shadow.

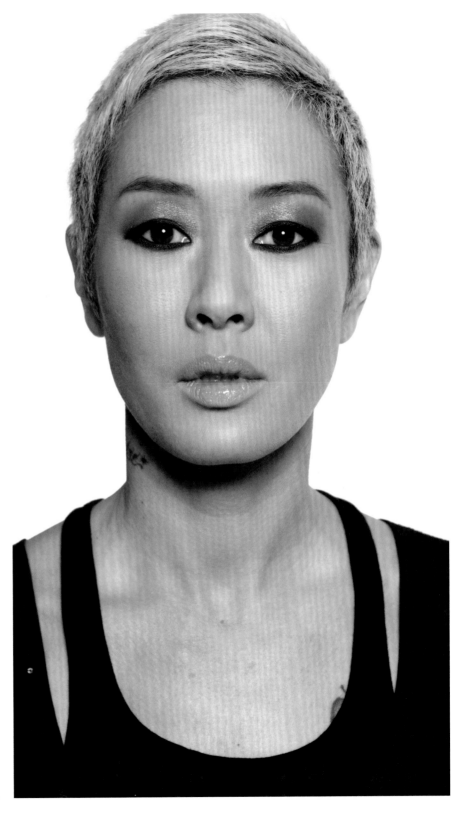

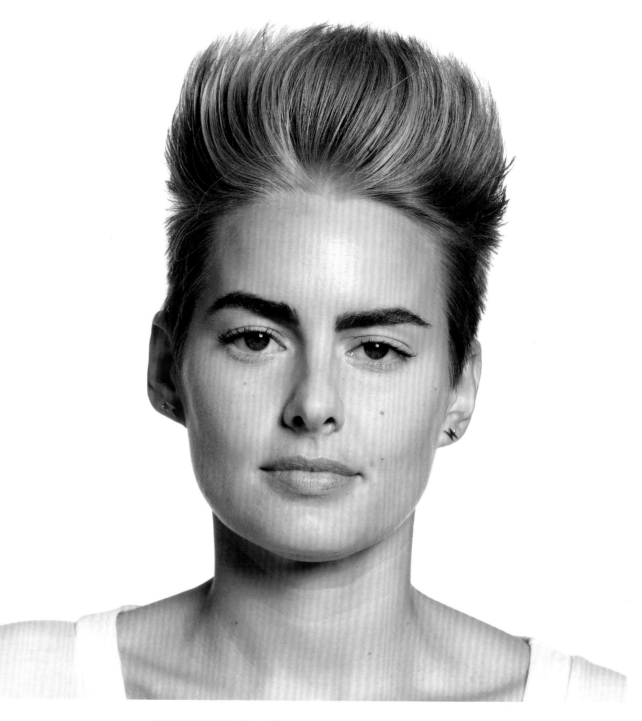

JENNIFER CROSS STUDIO MANAGER

My favorite makeup trick is putting clear mascara on eyebrows. It keeps them in the shape you desire.

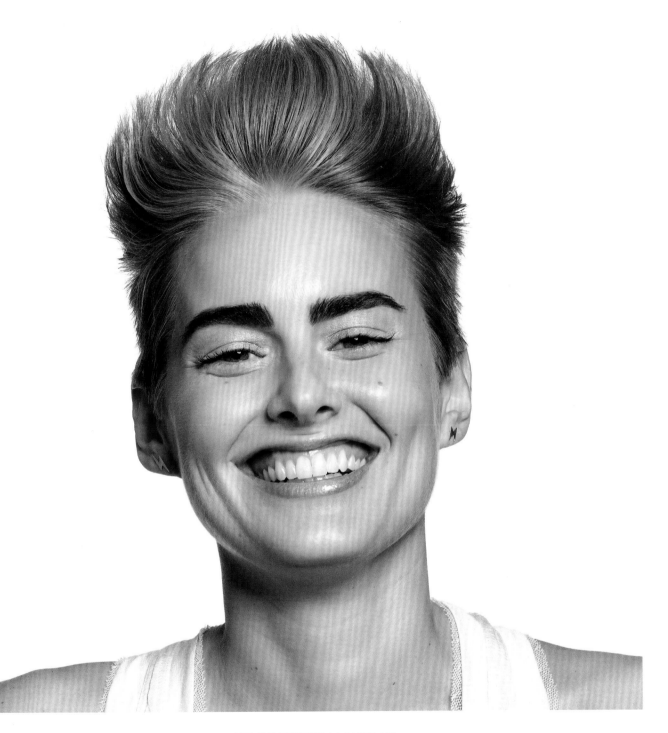

JENNIFER'S MAKEUP

Jennifer has striking brows, intense blue eyes, and a bold short cut—all of which command attention—so I kept the rest of her makeup soft and luminous. A pale yellow eye shadow topped with a champagne shimmer brightens up her eyes. I applied coral pot rouge on her cheeks highlighted with a coral shimmer blush on the cheekbones and added a peach lip gloss to give Jennifer an all-over glow.

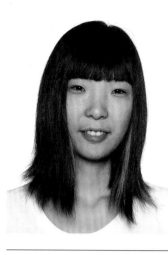

MAI KATO
GRAPHIC DESIGNER

I couldn't find meaning in my life for a long time. I compared myself to other people a lot, and I wanted to be somebody I was not. But at some point I realized that I have to live my life instead of somebody else's.

MAI'S MAKEUP—DAY

I love how Mai's bangs frame her stunning dark eyes. To highlight her eyes even more, I used a concealer brush with a peach corrector followed by a yellow-based creamy concealer to brighten undereye darkness. Ivory shadow on the lids, a thin line of black gel liner on the top lash line, and lengthening mascara complete this bold look.

MAI'S MAKEUP— NIGHT

I played up Mai's natural flush by sweeping pale pink blush on the apples of her cheeks. For a very subtle glow, I used a rose highlighter pen on her cheekbone. Ruby lips with a fresh face looks cool and modern.

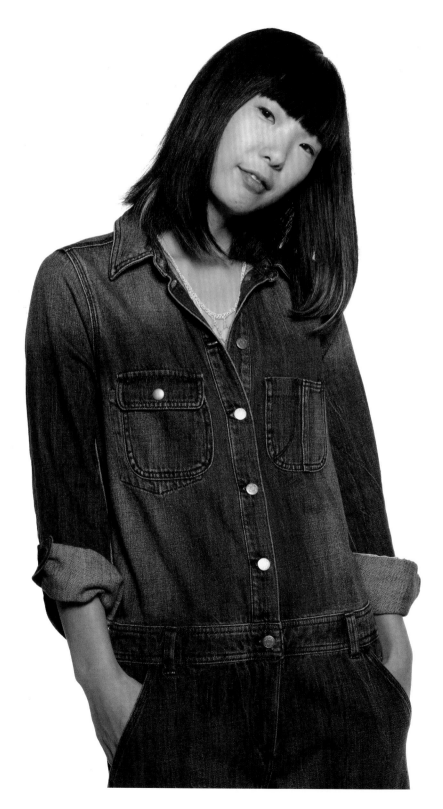

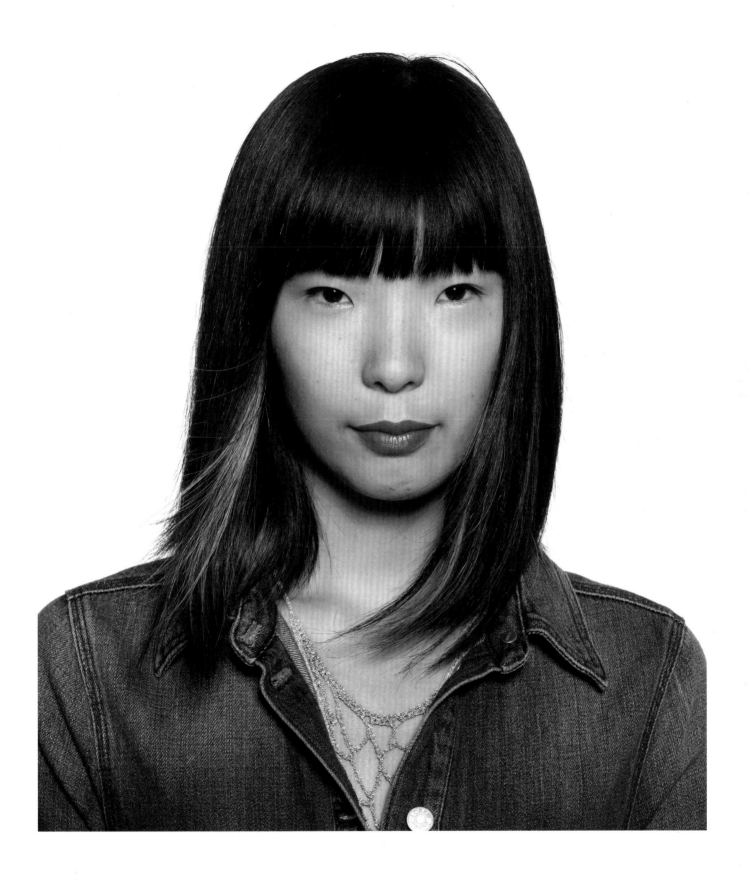

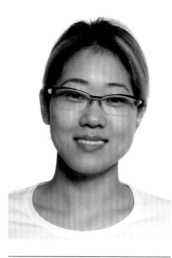

JULIA KIM
HAIRSTYLIST

I've discovered that black liquid eyeliner and mascara can turn your whole day (if not your whole outlook) around.

JULIA'S MAKEUP— DAY

From her clothes to her glasses to her hair, Julia exudes personality. I applied a light bronzer with a pop of a bright pink blush to bring a warm healthy color to Julia's face. A beige lip color with a touch of beige gloss gives Julia an understated yet cool look that complements her hip sense of style.

JULIA'S MAKEUP— NIGHT

In the evening, switch your glasses for contacts and accentuate your eyes with a thick line of black gel liner. For a luminescent glow, I gave Julia an additional sweep of peony blush on her cheeks followed with a rose highlighter on the cheekbones. The vivid hot pink lip gives Julia a confident, flirty pout.

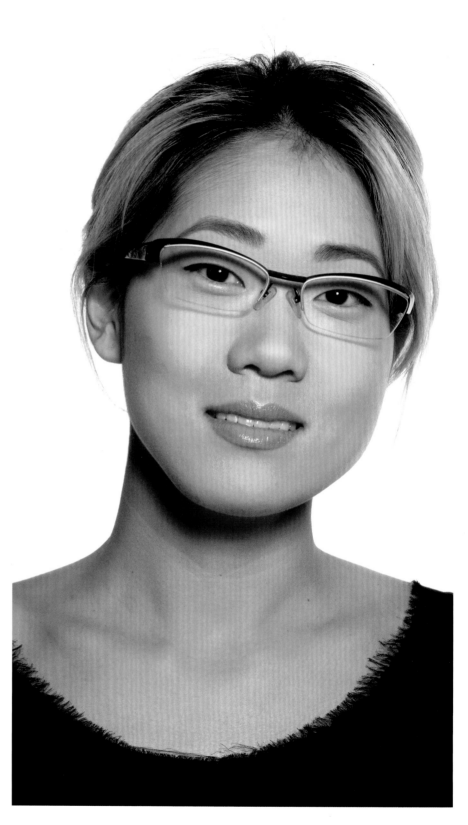

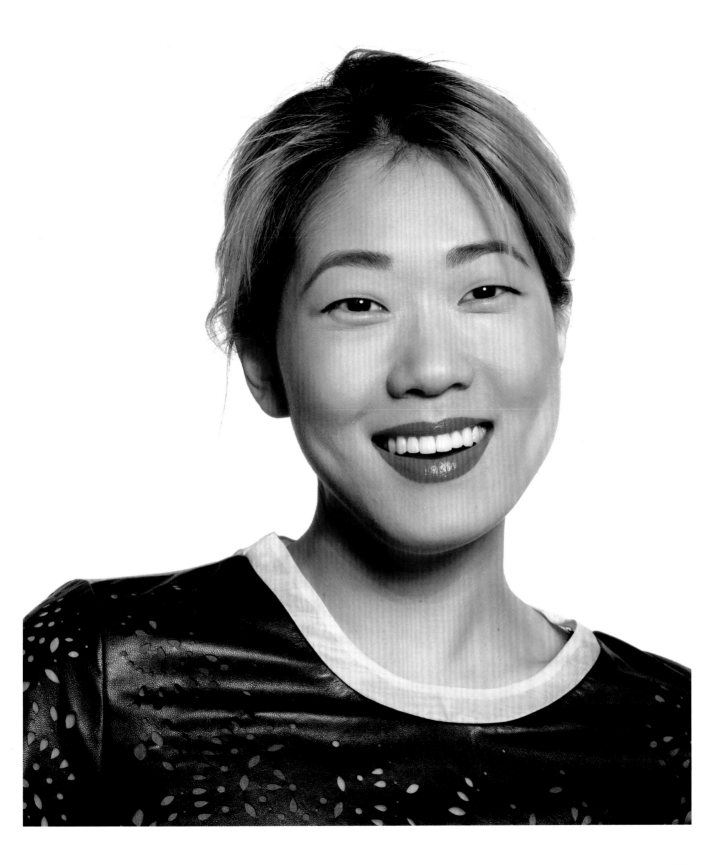

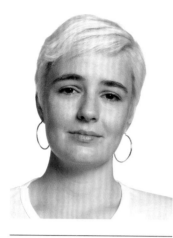

JOLIE WERNETTE-HORN MAGAZINE ART DIRECTOR

I love my eyes. They are so dark and expressive. I like that my dyed platinum hair makes them seem even bolder.

JOLIE'S MAKEUP

I really like the contrast between a polished bright red lip and platinum hair. The pop of red looks very contemporary and pretty on Jolie. A coral shimmer blush adds a subtle brightness to her face that enhances her gorgeous red lips.

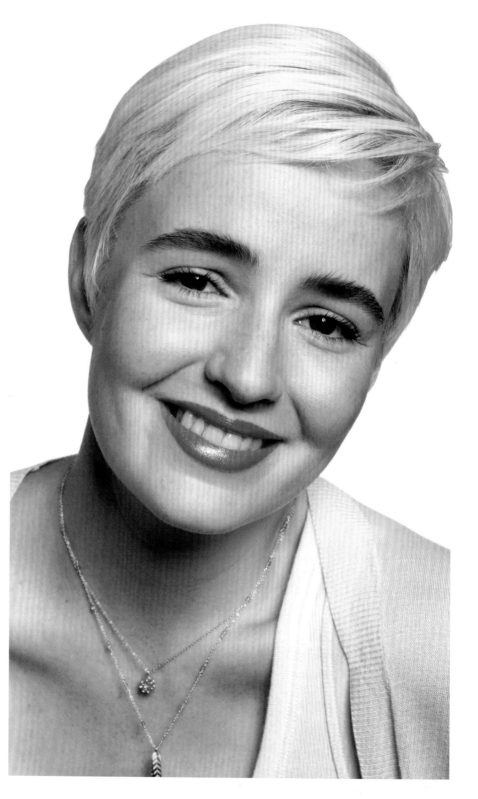

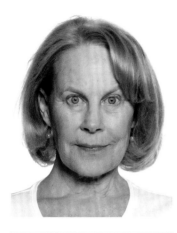

MARY ALICE WILLIAMS
BROADCAST JOURNALIST, COLLEGE PROFESSOR

I see the glass as half full. It's my stubborn, sturdy optimism that is the driving force behind everything that I do. I always look for the best in people and situations and believe there's a lesson to be found in every experience.

MARY ALICE'S MAKEUP

Mary Alice has dazzling blue-green eyes. To enhance this color, I relied on a very navy gel liner on top and a softer slate grey shadow on the lower rims. If you have fair lashes like Mary Alice, applying several coats of black volumizing mascara will lengthen and define lashes for a stunning look.

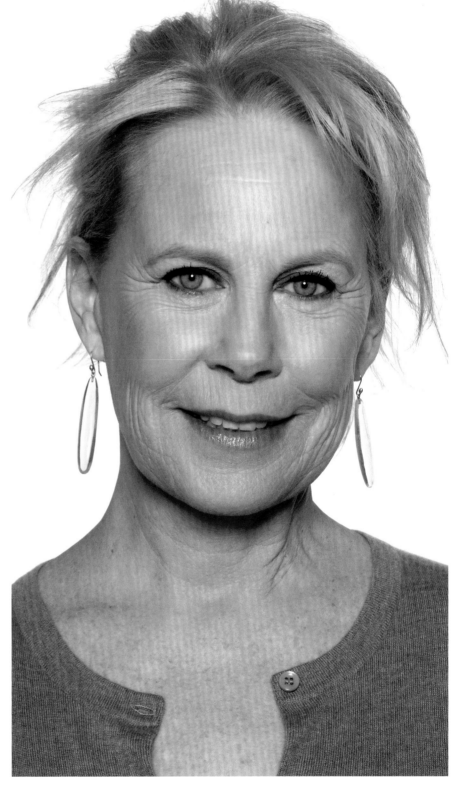

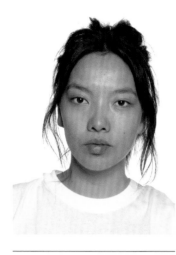

YESHE TENZIN GYALTAG
RESTAURANT MANAGER, MUSICIAN

I think pretty comes from the inside.

YESHE'S MAKEUP

Because Yeshe has her own cool standout sense of style, we didn't want to overdo her makeup. Sometimes being bold means less packs more punch. On Yeshe, a statement lip or a smoky eye would be too obvious and overpower her look. Instead, thick black liner winged out at the edges paired with a nude glittery gloss lets her downtown style sparkle.

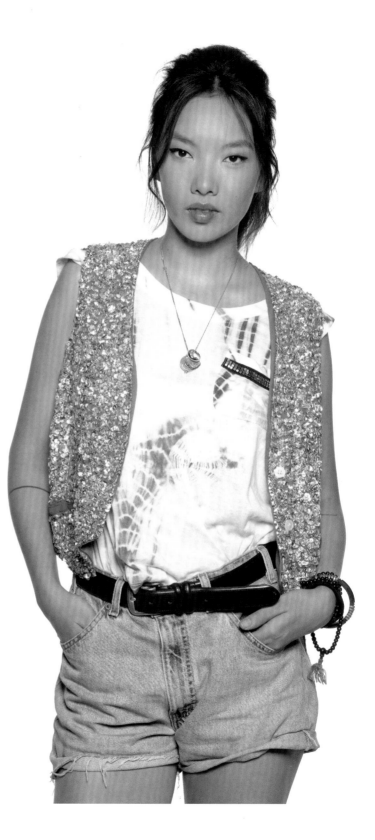

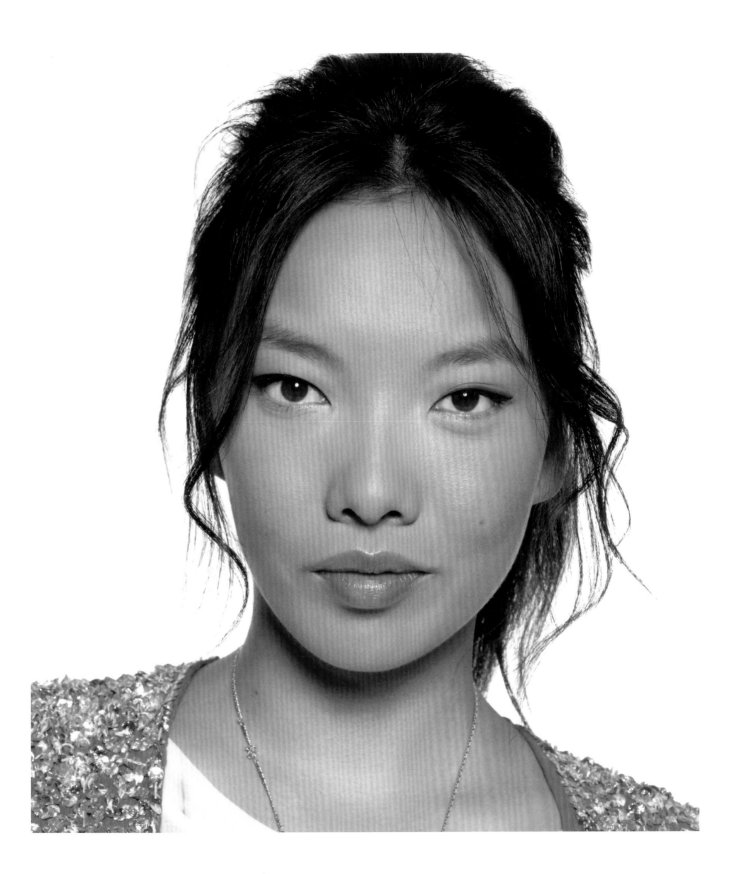

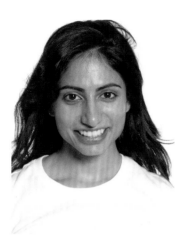

SUSIE ABRAHAM
FREELANCE
PUBLISHING
SPECIALIST

I wish I knew at fifteen to revel in your uniqueness. When you grow up in a place like Houston, Texas, and you want to look like a Southern belle but you don't, just learning to appreciate why you look different and why you are different is so important. Having a culture and identity makes you special.

SUSIE'S MAKEUP

To create Susie's gorgeous smoky eyes, I paired taupe and brown metallic shadows on her lids with charcoal and black liner. The combination of a beige lip with strong eyes is both sexy and modern.

EYELINER TIP

When you do an over-the-top smoky eye, it's important that you keep the liner on the lower rim very soft. You can accomplish this by using a long-wear eye pencil, applying it very close to the lashes, and smudging before it sets.

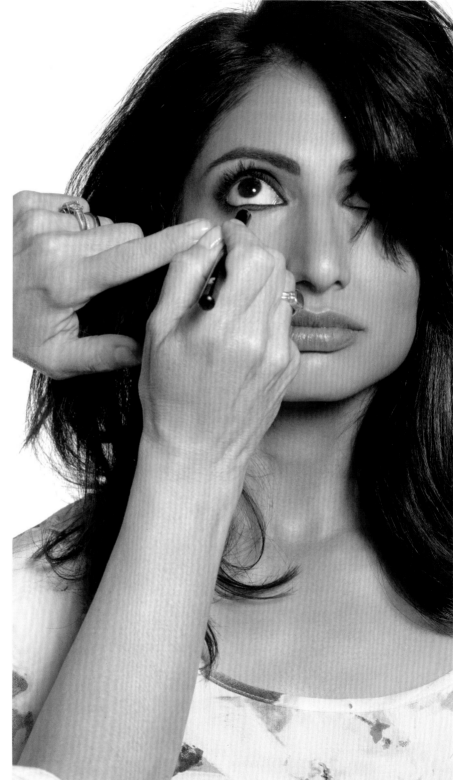

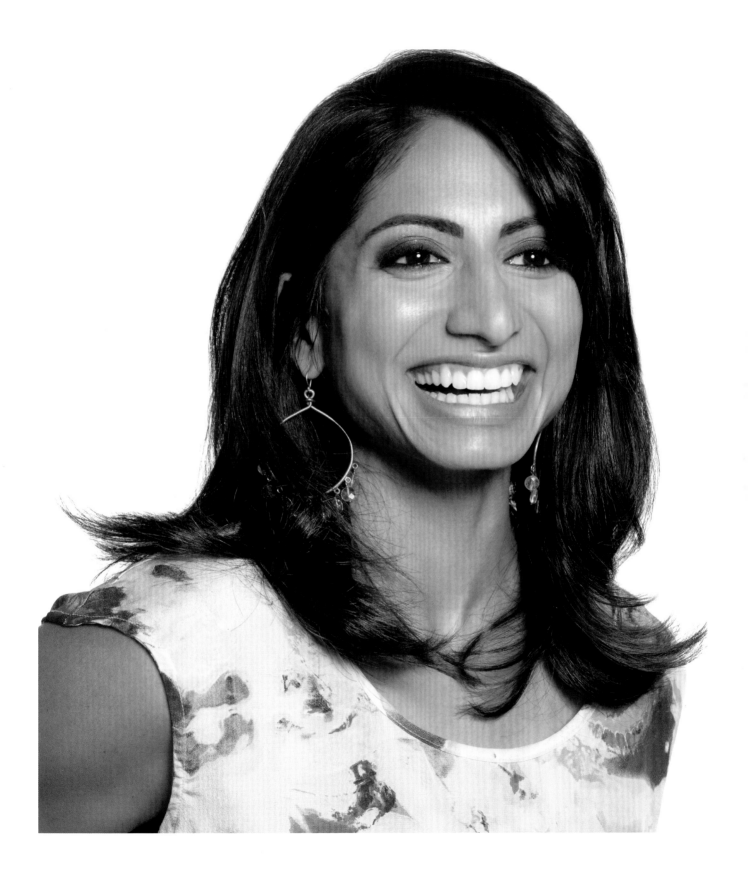

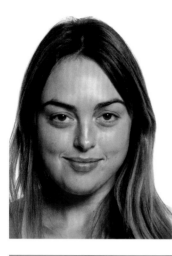

ALESSANDRA STEINHERR
MAGAZINE BEAUTY DIRECTOR

When I was young, I was convinced there was only one singular definition of beauty: tan, slim, and blonde. Now, as time passes, I've realized that there are so many kinds of beautiful, and I've never felt more confident in myself or my own unique looks.

ALESSANDRA'S MAKEUP

To give Alessandra a dramatic look, we focused on her stunning eyes and brows. To accentuate her naturally prominent brows, we brushed a mahogany shadow following her natural arch. For a soft sheen on lids, we applied a beige cream shadow all over. The wow factor was added with liner: A strong line of black-brown gel liner on her upper lash line and a dark brown shadow on the lower lash line create a wonderfully bold look.

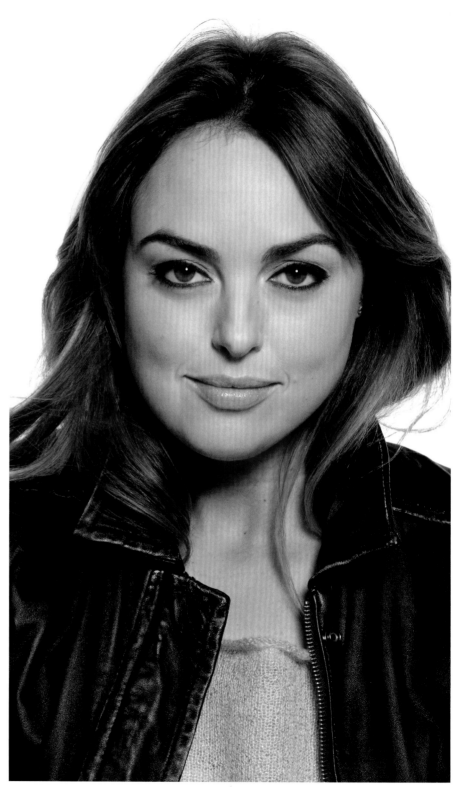

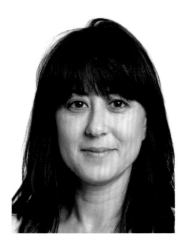

MIMI KOZMA
TEACHER

I can't live without mascara. Eyes speak volumes, and my eyes disappear without it.

MIMI'S MAKEUP

Mimi, who is one of my son's former teachers, usually wears very minimal makeup. For fun, we decided to give her a totally different look. Glamorous smoky eyes paired with sweet pink lips and cheeks showed Mimi how to be bold without looking over the top. It's important to play with your look. You never know what will bring you confidence.

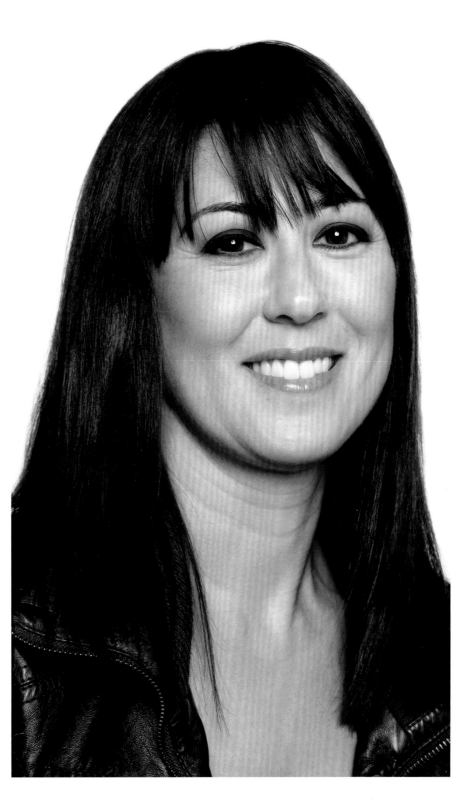

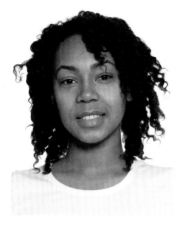

MUFFY GAYNOR
HIP-HOP
RECORDING ARTIST

I love to dance because it makes me feel truly free, like a bird that's just taken flight.

MUFFY'S MAKEUP— DAY

Muffy is a performer, and a silvery shimmer cream shadow makes Muffy's eyes light up and gives her a scene-stealing look. A bronzer with a bit of shimmer, a tawny blush, and a light beige gloss bring a subtle touch of color to her face while letting her eyes take center stage.

MUFFY'S MAKEUP— NIGHT

With the shimmery eyes, a bright fuchsia-pink lip color applied with a brush is all Muffy needs for a playful and bold nighttime look.

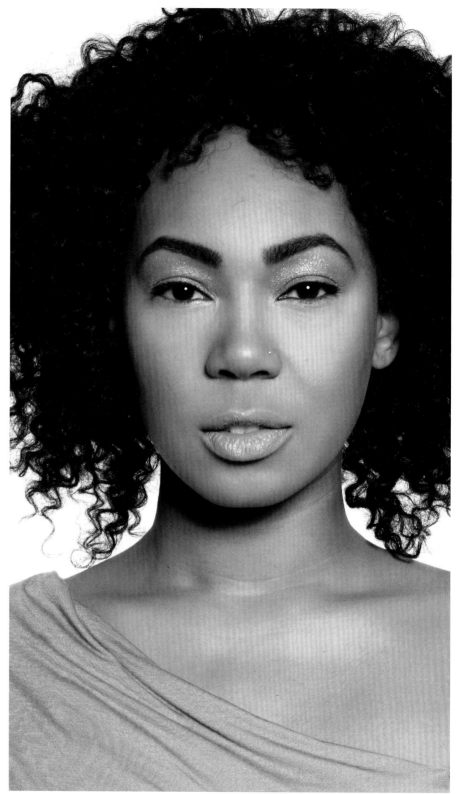

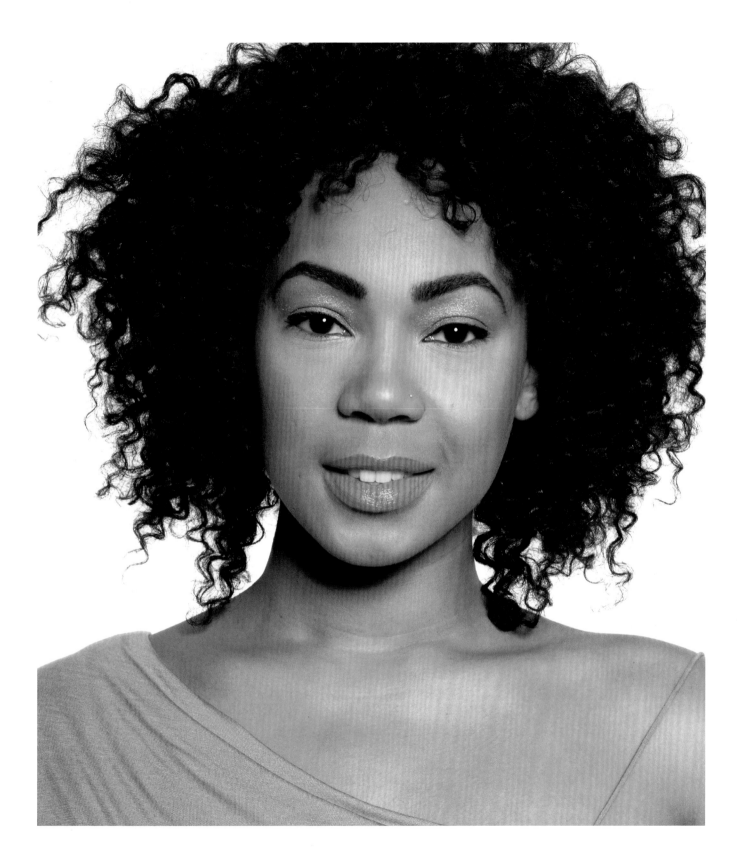

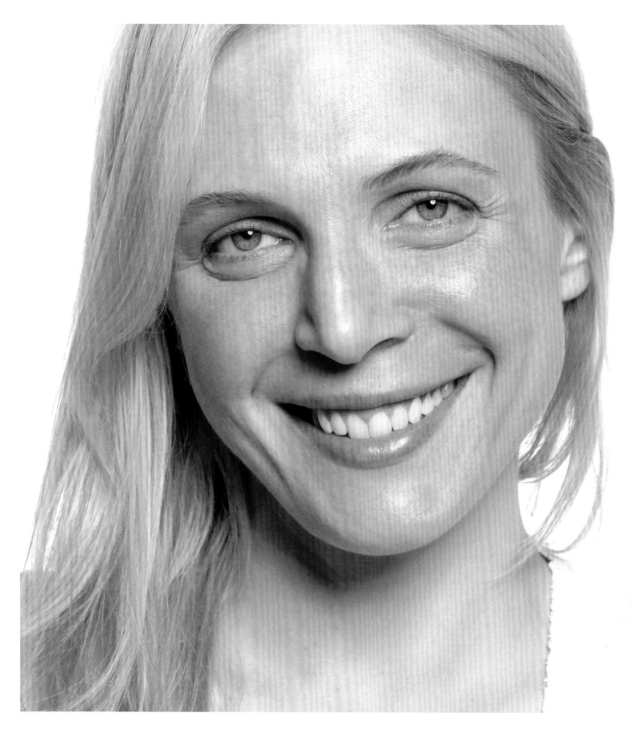

ANNABEL TOLLMAN FASHION STYLIST

I wish I'd had more courage and sort of lived on the edge a bit more. It sounds crazy because I've been quite brave in my life. But I wish I knew at eighteen that you can just walk up to people and say, "I really like what you do; I'd really like to work with you." Or that you can just know what you want to do and take positive steps rather than thinking, Oh, that's just a dream and I'll never do it.

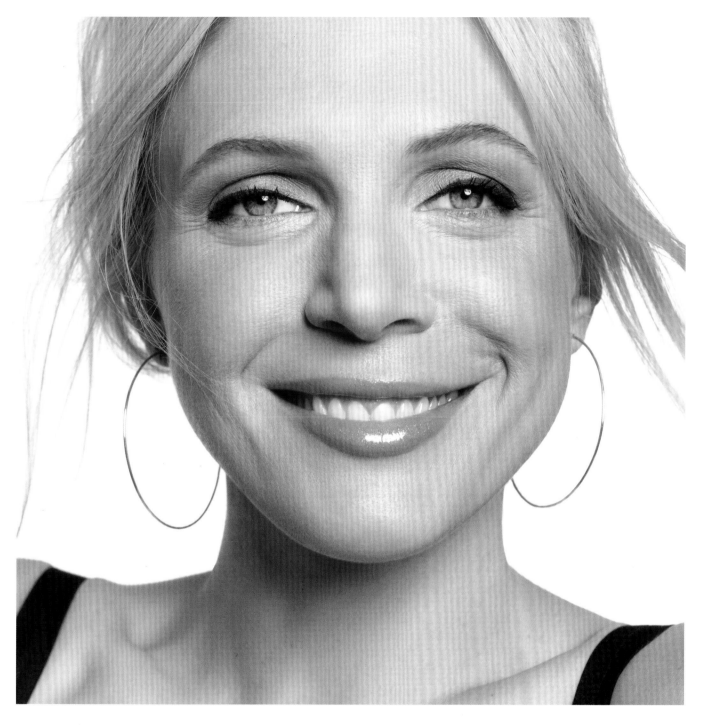

ANNABEL'S MAKEUP

When you have blue eyes and fair skin like Annabel, you want to use makeup to really define the eyes. A light touch of a medium gray-brown brow pencil adds depth to her eyebrows. On her lids, I layered a mix of beige and silvery-brown shimmer all over with a grayish-beige shadow in the crease. To bring out the blue in her eyes and create a sexy evening look, I went for a deep black-brown gel liner combined with navy and dark gray shadow liners smudged on top.

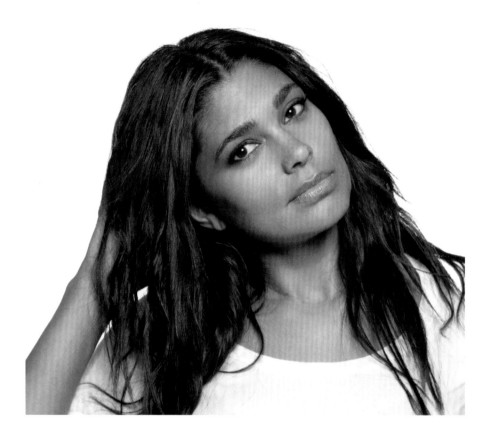

RACHEL ROY
FASHION DESIGNER

As a creative person, Rachel understands how to tap into personal expression. She lets her moods dictate her style, and she likes to change it up. I've seen her looking totally polished and uptown as well as edgy and downtown. Rachel is becoming an icon in the fashion world, but she is also a very involved and loving mom. She straddles the worlds of work and being a mom like I do, so we've had many of those *How do you do it?* talks. I've been doing the makeup for her runway shows since she launched her brand, and it's been amazing to watch her go after her dream and turn her business into a success.

—

Rachel loves to experiment with different looks through makeup. Because of her confidence, she can carry a smokier eye than most women, and the look suits her beautifully day or night. A black gel liner on the top lashes, kohl liner around the eyes, and charcoal shadow smudged on both top and bottom lids give Rachel showstopping eyes.

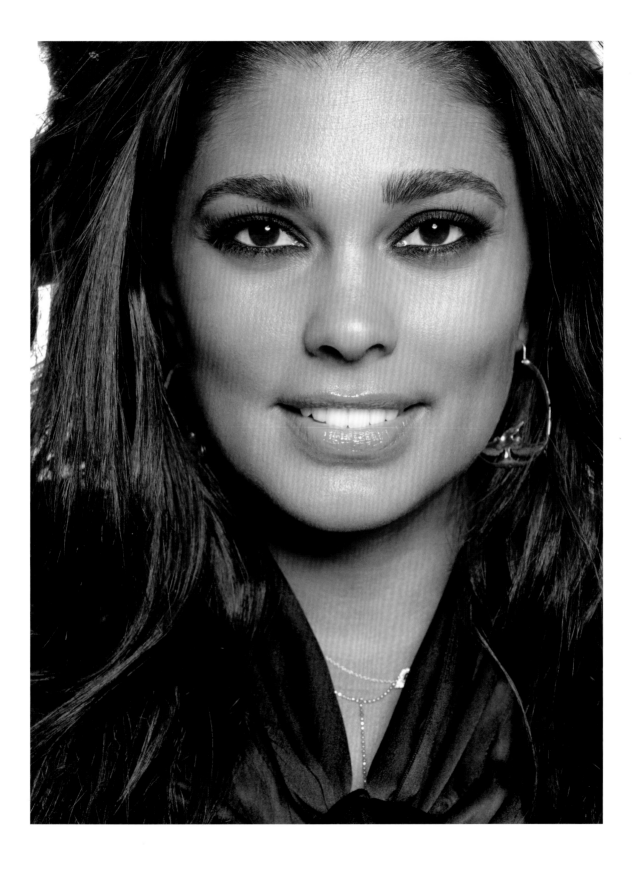

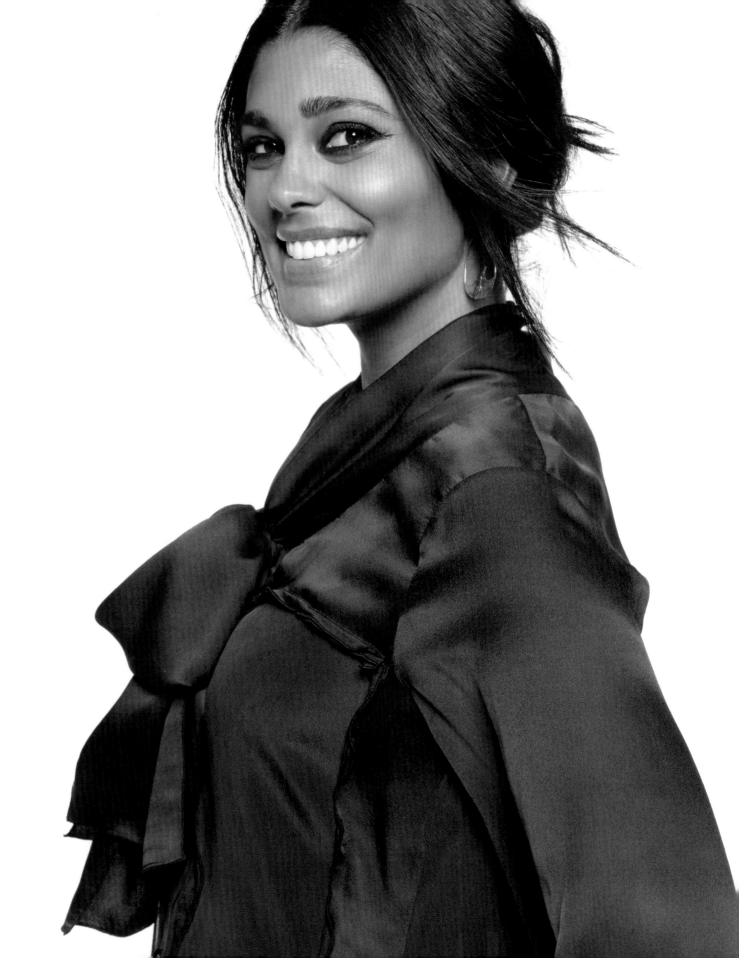

I love the feeling of accomplishing something that I have been told "no" about.

—RACHEL ROY

Without balance there is no happiness. You can work your tush off, but if you don't have a personal life or a love life—whether that is your children or your pets or your garden or however love comes to you—I don't think you'll be happy.

I feel pretty when someone that I love is looking at me with that look, where I can tell that they just think that I have it and that I can't be replaced. It might be my three-year-old looking at me when I have heels and a dress on, or my eleven-year-old when I have just accomplished something that in her mind is scary and I nail it, or a guy looking at me the way that I want him to.

I am trying my best to be the woman that I want my girls to be, and it is quite hard because I want to do it by actions and not by words.

I have had so many moments in my life where I didn't feel pretty, and if I go back to the source of why I didn't feel pretty, it was all about what was going on inside. So when I dress people, particularly young girls, I tell them that whatever they think about themselves is what someone else will think about them. I know it is really hard to grasp and it sounds corny, but it really is true. So however I'm feeling on the inside, I try to tell the story on the outside through hair, makeup, and clothing.

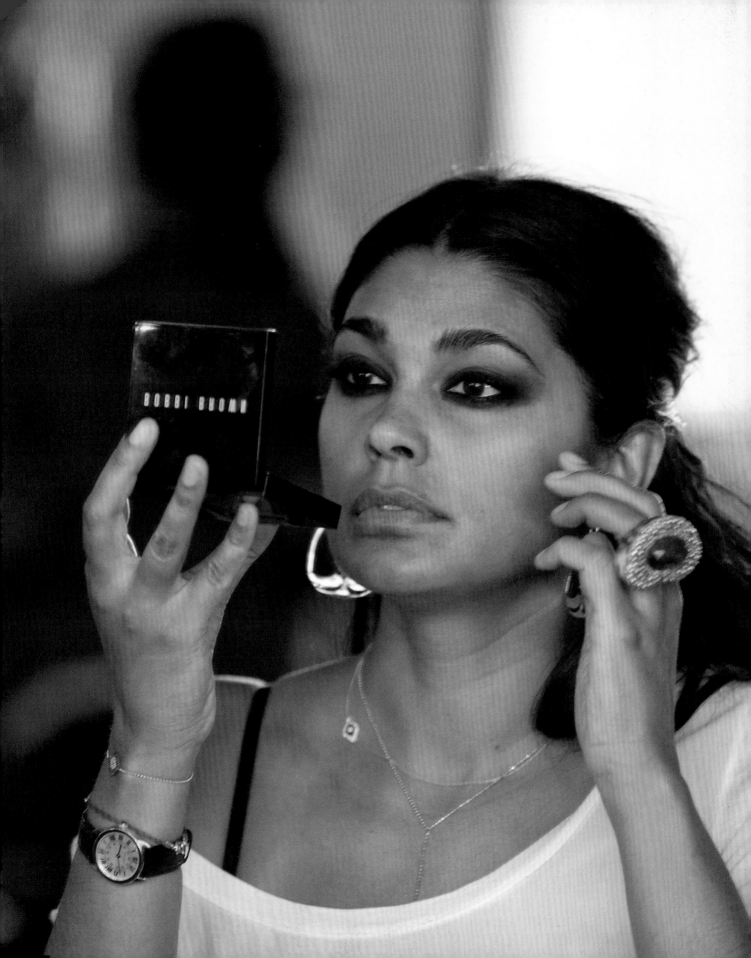

Knowing what you can do at any given time to look and feel better is pretty powerful.

—BOBBI BROWN

SURPRISE YOURSELF

Getting out of your comfort zone

———

Women look and feel their best when they are comfortable. But if you don't experiment with different looks, you can get stuck in a beauty rut. You will never know what looks, colors, or formulas you will fall in love with unless you try them.

PRETTY NATURAL

Play with texture. Don't be afraid of shimmer, glimmer, matte, shine, or gloss. While you can experiment with texture in the colors you are comfortable with, don't shy away from makeup colors that don't look like you. Try one pop of something a little brighter or bolder with your regular makeup.

PRETTY RADIANT

Try any look, because you can. Go for the most natural simple makeup, with sheer gloss, clear balm on lids, soft cheeks, and a sweep of mascara. Or go over-the-top bold and funky with edgy eyes or look-at-me bright lips. Just make sure your makeup has shine to it; illuminating formulas always work for you.

PRETTY STRONG

Go glam. Ditch the yoga pants and fleece and show off those toned legs and arms. Go for a strong eye, a thicker sweep of gel eyeliner, or a classic red lip. Going from sporty to a chic, polished Grace Kelly or Jackie O look could feel new and fresh.

PRETTY CLASSIC

Try not to be so perfect and put together. That doesn't mean letting go completely; just try to do something that's not so polished. Smudge your eyeliner, take a break from the lip liner, and dab on a pot rouge straight from the pot. Experiment with less makeup—nothing on eyes but mascara, a lighter foundation, or a very soft blush.

PRETTY AUTHENTIC

To break up your beauty routine, try a completely of-the-moment trend—feathers, a different hemline, the color of the season. Whether it is blue nails, the red lip you've always wanted to try, or a plunging neckline, play with a totally new look and see how it feels.

PRETTY BOLD

Going with understated, subtle makeup is another way to surprise people. It is also a way to let your authentic natural beauty shine through. For example, I think Lady Gaga looks the most beautiful and stunning when she has a bare face. It's like she is taking off her mask and revealing herself a bit more.

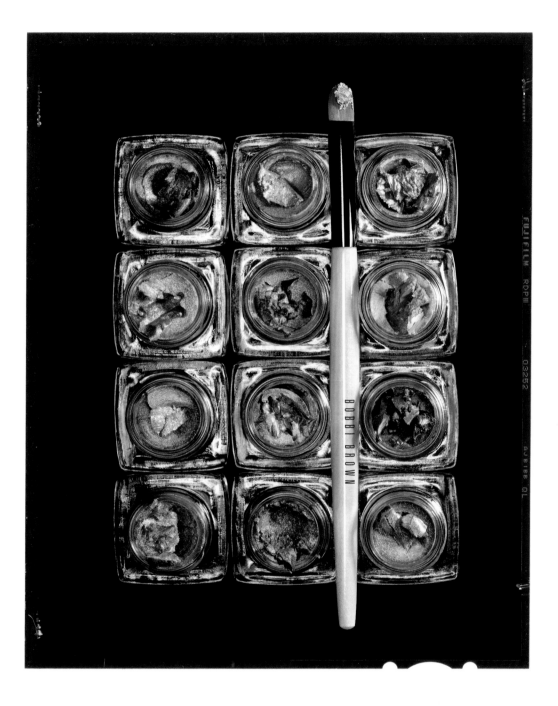

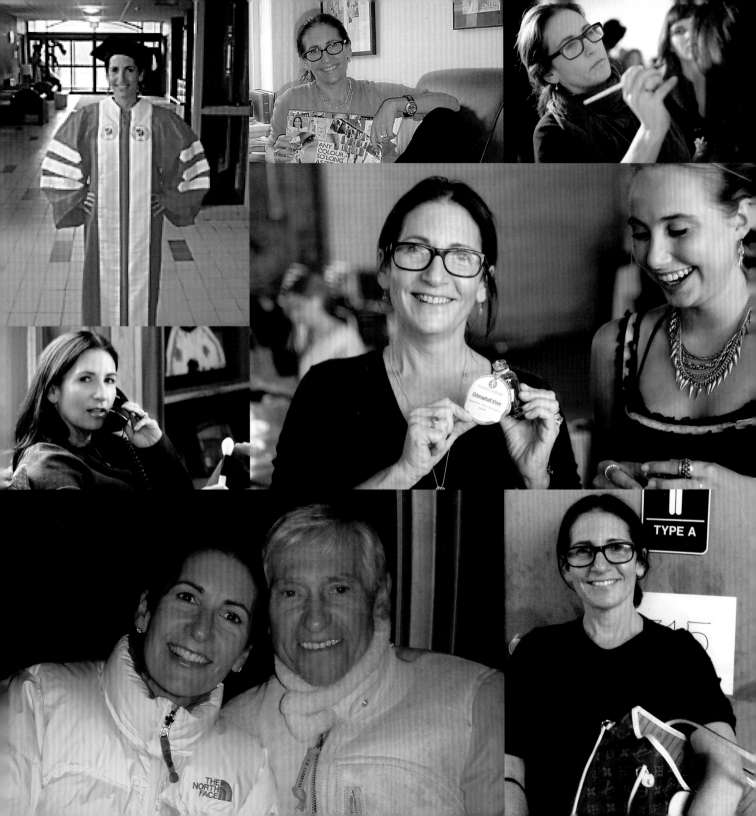

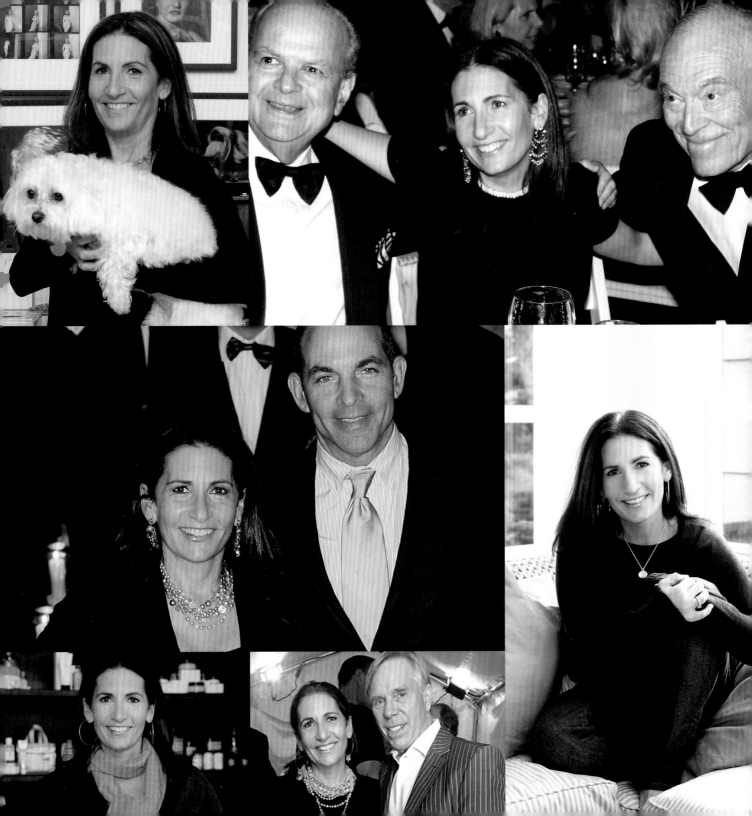

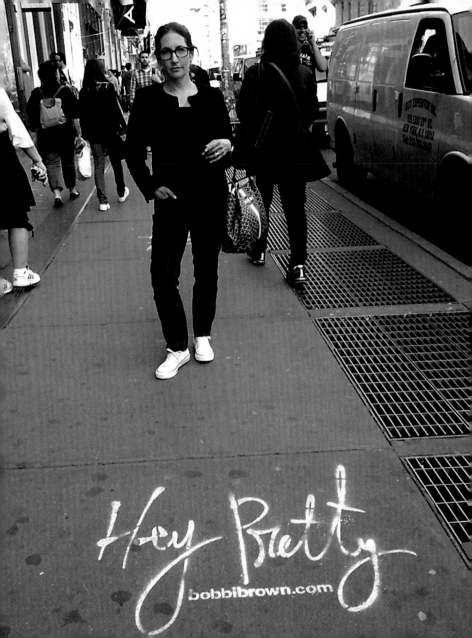

My Bobbi Brown makeup artists, who are always pretty powerful to me—Kimberly Soane, Marc Reagan, Ricki Gurtman, Cassandra Garcia, Kai Vinson, Elizabeth Keiser, Tanya Cropsey, Hannah Martin, Laramie Glen, and Lindsey Jones. Eric Dominguez and Carlos Martin, for their constant support and ability to create effortless hair. Kim Colville, my amazing stylist, who can do it all—from organizing booking to shopping and styling—she was the tough, funny glue that held the shoot together. My New York Bobbi team—Donald Robertson, Alicia Sontag, Ruba Abu-Nimah, Lahnie Strange, Eleanor Rogers, Kevin Ley, MC Katigbak, Roza Israel, Jen Pountain, and Kate Wyman—I am so grateful for your creative visions and support. To my unstoppable PR team—Veronika Ullmer, Alexis Rodriguez, Corinne Zadigan, and Gretchen Berra—you rule!

To my wonderful publishing team at Chronicle Books, led by Christine Carswell—Aya Akazawa, Jennifer Tolo Pierce, Tera Killip, Laura Lee Mattingly, Liza Algar, Claire Fletcher, and Doug Ogan.

And to all the inspiring Pretty Powerful women—my heartfelt thanks goes out to you.

CREDITS

___

PROJECT MANAGEMENT

Jill Cohen

Kim Colville

Samantha Kopf

PHOTOGRAPHY

Ondrea Barbe

Ian Gipe – Agent

Justin Francavilla – First Assistant

Alex Yerks – Digital Technician

Ben Ritter

Henry Leutwyler

BOBBI BROWN MONTCLAIR, NEW JERSEY STUDIO

Ralph Izzard

Michael Cisneros

Florenz Paredes

Danielle Lopes

Susana Canario

Yuby Leoce

INDUSTRIA

Fabrizio Ferri

Stephanie Wilson

FILM/VIDEO

Dickie Plofker – director

Andy Garland – Producer/DP

Brian Johnson – Production Manager

Pedro Pacilla – Camera operator

Shane Duckworth – Alexa AC

Brian Parrish – Production coordinator

Matt Tomko – Gaffer

Eric Hora – Electric

Ssong Yang – Grip

Charles Cann – Sound

Davis Northern – PA Driver

Biliana Starcevic – Stand In

MAKEUP ARTISTS

Kimberly Soane

Elizabeth Keiser

Ricki Gurtman

Cassandra Garcia

Kai Vinson

Marc Reagan

Tanya Cropsey

Hannah Martin

Laramie Glen

Lindsey Jones

CATERING

Uptown Restaurant Montclair

D'Orazio Catering

HAIR

Eric Dominguez

Lauren Gensinger

MANICURIST

Roza Israel

DRIVERS

Ron Hill

Crestwood

Tyler Drewitz

STYLISTS

Gabi Dolce-Bengtsson

Elizabeth Cohen

Cathleen Donohue

CLOTHING

White + Warren

Spanx

Gryphon New York

MODELS

Lauren Bush

Abby Stedman

Kirby Bumpus

Gabrielle Nevin

April Perry

Marie Clare Katigbak

Jay Golson

Sarah Carden

Cindi Leive

Gabourey Sidibe

Alexis Rodriguez

Lee Heh Margolies

Gro Frivoll

Janice Chou

Susana Canario

Alexis Stewart

Erica Reid

Tina Craig

Eva Pichardo

Alyssa Hulahan

Rosanne Guararra

Alexa Ray Joel

Keisher McLeod-Wells

Teisher McLeod

Alana Monique Beard

Danielle Diamond

Jennifer Kohl

Crystal Gaynor

Angel Williams

Cristie Kerr

Natalie Gulbis

Laurel Wassner

Rebeccah Wassner

Nancy Donahue

Jacquie Antinoro

Saskia Miller

Alexandra Wilson

Alexis Maybank

Perivush Shahzad

Laurel Pantin

Denise Johnson

Hannah Martin

Jo-Ann Howe

Alexandra Brazier

Anne Gimm Naughton

Blythe Danner

Lee Woodruff

Sue Torres

Granvilette Kestenbaum

Lauren Kestenbaum

Sara Blakely

Lauren Rifkin

Beth Baldwin

Liz Murray

Rose Cali

Sarma Melngailis

Sandra Bernhard

Estelle

Jenny Shimizu

Jennifer Cross

Mai Kato

Julia Kim

Jolie Wernette-Horn

Mary Alice Williams

Yeshe Tenzin Gyaltag

Susie Abraham

Alessandra Steinherr

Mimi Kozma

Muffy Gaynor

Annabel Tollman

Rachel Roy

INDEX

———

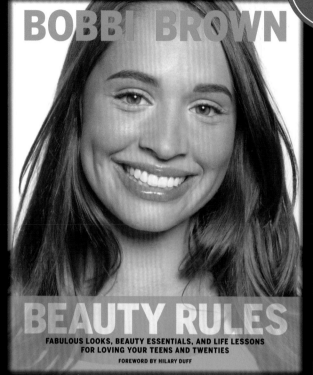

Also from bestselling author and famed makeup artist Bobbi Brown comes this definitive beauty book empowering teens and twenty-somethings with age-appropriate makeup tips, style secrets, and self-esteem boosters. Emphasizing natural beauty, Bobbi advises on the best products and tools for keeping skin of every type flawless, and shares step-by-step techniques for getting the prettiest hair, eyes, lips, and nails. Stunning makeovers inspire looks for school, parties, interviews, and beyond. With hundreds of photos of real girls, shots of celebrity role models, and Bobbi's best tricks from her remarkable career in the cosmetics industry, *Beauty Rules* is the go-to guide for all girls.

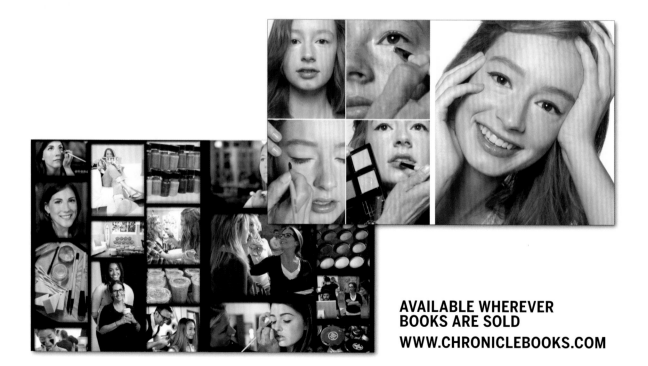